DISCARD
W9-BCD-106
South Haverhill Road
El Dorado, Kansas 67042-3280

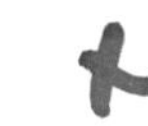

Mismanaged CARE

Mismanaged CARE

How Corporate Medicine Jeopardizes Your Health

MICHAEL E. MAKOVER, M.D.

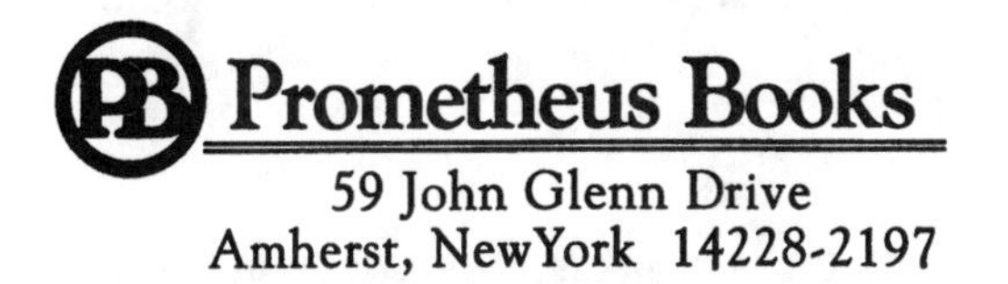
Prometheus Books
59 John Glenn Drive
Amherst, NewYork 14228-2197

Published 1998 by Prometheus Books

 Inquiries should be addressed to Prometheus Books, 59 John Glenn Drive, Amherst, New York 14228–2197, 716–691–0133. FAX: 716–691–0137. WWW.PROMETHEUSBOOKS.COM

02 01 00 99 98 5 4 3 2 1

Library of Congress Cataloging-in-Publication Data

Makover, Michael E.
Mismanaged care : how corporate medicine jeopardizes your health / by Michael E. Makover.
p. cm.
Includes bibliographical references and index.
ISBN 1–57392–248–X (cloth : alk. paper)
1. Managed care plans (Medical care)—United States. 2. Managed care plans (Medical care)—Moral and ethical aspects—United States. 3. Physician and patient—United States. 4. Medical care—United States—Finance. I. Title.
RA413.5.U5M33 1998
362.1'04258'0973—dc21 98–38860
CIP

Printed in the United States of America on acid-free paper.

To my father, Henry B. Makover, M.D.,
who taught me by his example, wisdom, and love
what a great doctor and a great father is.

To my mother, Mickey Makover,
who taught me by her example and love what great writing is
and how to approach life positively with joy and enthusiasm.

To my lovely wife, Terry,
whose love, support, and patience made this book possible.

To my children, Matthew and Heather,
who make every day special and wonderful.

To my brother, Richard B. Makover, M.D.,
whose wisdom, love, and support have always been invaluable.

Contents

Preface

This book is my own personal view. It is based on over thirty years of experience in medicine and extensive research by interview and by studying the available literature. I do not represent any organization. On the contrary, my purpose is to represent the interests of patients and their doctors. This book is designed for all who have been, are, or will be patients needing care.

There is enough written about health care to fill a library. There are enough viewpoints to fuel a thousand debates. I have not attempted to reproduce or cover all of that vast range of information.

Instead, my purpose is to present the issues that you must consider as you make your own choices in the area of health care.

This book is meant to be short, accessible, and useful. I have noted references where appropriate and have appended a glossary and a bibliography for those who need clarification or who want to read further. Obviously, a book such as this can become dated very quickly, so I have created a website (www.makover.com) to provide the most current information on health care in general and managed care in particular.

When individual cases that are not already published elsewhere are being discussed, I have altered enough identifying features to protect the privacy of the subjects of the story, but in no way have I distorted the relevant meaning.

I have avoided a long series of anecdotes and horror stories. A few are included to illustrate my point here and there, but anecdotes do not prove anything. What I have done instead is to attempt to meld logic and experience to stimulate fresh thinking on these subjects.

I speak my views quite forthrightly and I expect to be the target of those I criticize. I have done so because I believe someone must stand up and speak for the disenfranchised of today's medical world: the patients and those doctors who are trying to preserve ethical, high-quality medicine in the face of great adversity.

At many points, you will find critical remarks about bureaucrats, politicians, businesspersons, and lawyers. I do *not* think these are bad people and there is *no* conspiracy of any kind that is responsible for the problems I identify. *Even if each person performs his or her individual functions exactly as he or she should, the problem is the process, not the people.*

The doctors, nurses, and executives of managed care companies are another matter. You will have to judge for yourself whether they are making socially valuable business decisions or whether they are making self-serving rationalizations to justify the enormous amounts of money they receive while denying so much to so many, often with significant harm.

I believe that current health care economics violate vital basic medical ethics.

We need better answers to our problems. Whatever they may be, they *must* be ethical.

We must not sacrifice our principles for expediency, for that will not only cost us more money in the end, it will cost us our souls as well.

Michael E. Makover, M.D.
New York
August 18, 1998

Acknowledgments

Many people contributed to the development of the ideas in this book and to bringing it to fruition. Unfortunately, I cannot list them all here.

In my research for this book, I have spoken to hundreds of physicians and many others in other disciplines of medicine and in business, far too many to list here. My thanks to them all.

(Some physicians asked to remain anonymous because they genuinely feared that being associated with a book critical of managed care could cause them problems in their dealings with the managed care companies. This fact alone is a condemnation of the managed care industry. That senior practitioners in America are fearful of speaking what they believe is a little chilling.)

The Hon. Jed Rakoff, Federal District Judge, was extremely helpful in areas related to the law.

I greatly appreciate the assistance of Robert Downey, a limited partner of Goldman, Sachs, who was of great assistance concerning business and financial questions.

I am very greatful to Richard Thau, Executive Director of Third Millennium (a nonprofit advocacy group for the rights of younger people), who believed in my project and brought the book to the publisher. He has been a valuable source of information, editing, and advice.

I am very appreciative of my editor, Steven L. Mitchell, COO, VP, and Editor-in-Chief of Prometheus Books. He has been very supportive and helpful throughout and has made many valuable suggestions. Assistant editor Kathy Deyell contributed many additional helpful suggestions and put great effort into preparing the manuscript for publication.

Samuel Packer, M.D., an experienced practicing clinician who has also held many leadership positions in medical organizations, has made important contributions in this field and was very generous in sharing his ideas and his own extensive library of resource materials.

The legal department of the Medical Society of the State of New York was very helpful in supplying legal resources.

I extend my appreciation to my agents, Bill Adler and Tracy Quinn of Adler & Robin Books, who helped complete negotiations.

My thanks to *U.S. News & World Report* for permission to use quotations from "What Is the Value of a Voice," copyright March 9, 1998, *U.S. News & World Report.*

My wife, Terry, has made many valuable suggestions. This book was written with a very tight deadline, which necessitated long stretches of intensive work. I could not have succeeded without the help of my wife and children, who put in great effort to make that possible and very generously put up with my being locked to my word processor for so many hours.

We physicians learn most from one source—our patients. It is with great appreciation that I thank all the thousands of patients I have seen over the past thirty-four years and from whom I have received so much in return.

Prologue

The Rationale for the Managed Care Revolution

A true revolution has occurred in the financing of health care in America. Since 1990, managed care, which had been evolving slowly over a long time, came to totally dominate and change health care in this country.

In the 1970s and 1980s, health costs rose rapidly, especially for hospital care and procedures. The use of expensive procedures escalated rapidly, as did the fees charged for them. There seemed to be little incentive to control costs, limit hospital stays, or question procedures as long as insurance companies simply passed along the cost increases to employers. Corporations began to experience increased financial drains from the rapidly increased cost of paying for health coverage for their employees. Individuals who paid for their own insurance or who contributed to their health care premiums through payroll deductions likewise began to experience painful increases.

Managed care utilizes direct insurance as an alternative to indemnity insurance. As we will see in more detail later, indemnity insurance simply reimburses patients for bills submitted. On the other hand, direct insurers in effect hire doctors, hospitals, and other services to provide care to their subscribers, who pay the insurers to use those services. This critical difference gives the insurance company direct control over those providing health care to subscribers. This control allows the insurer to select doctors, hospitals, and other services; to control costs; to monitor what is being done; to attempt to measure the value of what is being done; and to enforce standards that it sets.

A central concept was that simple principles of sound business management should be applied to health care just as they are to every other business. Procedures and treatments should be tested to see if they actually produce the desired results, and only those that show value should be endorsed. Expensive experimental procedures—such as bone marrow transplants—were questioned since their value had not yet been conclusively proven.

It was widely believed that there were many medical procedures that continued to be used despite serious question as to their value, and others that were done in excess of real need. For example, it was observed that the frequency of operations such as coronary bypass surgery and caesarian deliveries varied widely by locality, although the patients seemed the same. Why would patients in one city need more bypass surgery than identical patients in another city? Either one place was doing too little or the other was doing too many. The conclusion was usually that there were too many surgeries.

Other health care techniques, such as preventive medicine, were being underutilized.

Obviously, prevention of problems is preferable to having to treat them. Vaccination rates were low in most places, many women did not get prenatal care that might identify or even avoid some problems, and many children did not get frequent enough well-child check-ups for preventive purposes. Mammograms to detect early stages of breast cancer seemed to be used far less frequently than they should have been.

Another perceived problem was that patients' care was too often fragmented as they went from specialist to specialist with no one coordinating their care. It was also thought that specialists were too expensive to treat many problems that general doctors could have handled. It was perceived that patients of specialists underwent many more procedures and surgeries than those of primary care doctors. Not only was this expensive, there were those who thought that the procedures were excessive and unnecessary and were detrimental to the patients.

Hospital care is extremely expensive. Routine stays can cost thousands of dollars per day. Intensive care and other specialized services are even more costly. Even empty hospital beds are expensive as they must be maintained in readiness. Throughout the 1970s and 1980s, the number of empty hospital beds was increasing steadily as hospitals continued to build and expand, seemingly oblivious to need. It was common knowledge that hospitals charged private patients at much higher rates than necessary in order to use the excess to finance the cost of medical research, medical education, and the care of the poor and uninsured. Some of these charges were so high that they raised the same kind of outcry as fifty-dollar nails did in the military. Despite the high costs, patients' hospital stays were not limited, and there was much time spent recovering in the hospital that could have been done at home or in less expensive facilities and while waiting for disposition to long-term care facilities like nursing homes. The hospitals had little incentive to control costs until Medicare changed how it reimbursed hospitals. Under the new method, Medicare no longer reimbursed hospital bills. Instead, the hospital was paid a set amount by Medicare for each diagnosis or group of diagnoses (DRGs, Diagnosis Related Groups), regardless of what it actually cost the hospital to provide the care. While some private insurers for non-Medicare patients began to make similar plans, in general this cost control feature applied only to Medicare patients.

The premiums for traditional insurance were rising far in excess of inflation. Total expenditures for health care began to consume a steadily higher percentage of the country's spending, reaching nearly 14 percent of the Gross Domestic Product (GDP). The projections were that health care expenditure would continue to rise until it represented more than 19 percent of the GDP by the year 2000.

As health care premiums increased, more and more Americans could no longer afford coverage and fewer small companies offered it as an employee benefit. The number of uninsured steadily increased.

Some of this has changed dramatically since managed care became the dominant force in health care financing. Hospital stays are now very brief for most conditions and a large percentage of inpatient procedures has been shifted to less expensive day-surgery facilities (where the patient is not admitted to the hospital and returns home on the same day) or to doctors' offices. Hospitals have closed whole wings, plans for building have been curtailed, and hospitals have merged into ever-larger conglomerates to achieve the cost efficiencies associated with size.

Doctors' fees are a small fraction of what they were previously, procedures are performed less often, and the costs of ancillary services such as laboratory tests, X-rays, and the like have been reduced.

Managed care companies require all patients to have a primary care doctor who coordinates their care and is the first doctor they see whenever something is wrong. Specialist referrals are now limited and can only be ordered by the primary doctor. Many procedures and visits must first be screened by the insurer's agents to ensure that they are appropriate and cost-effective. The insurers now monitor everything and use standardized measures of effectiveness and quality control. Doctors are screened before being allowed to participate in managed care plans and are held accountable for their performance. The insurers set standards for preventive care and monitor their doctors' compliance. Preventive care such as mammographies and vaccinations has increased among managed care patients.

Some managed care plans put the financial risk on the doctors by paying them a set amount per patient regardless of what the care costs. This, they feel, spurs the doctors to find innovative new ways to keep those patients healthier, since healthier patients cost less and thus mean more profit for the doctor.

Insurance premiums remained stable for a long time. Although increases are now occurring for the first time, they are still far below the rate of increase under the old system. Total health care expenditures for the country as a whole have now remained at about 14 percent of GDP for many years, contrary to the predictions that would have had it at 18 percent by the late 1990s.

Patients no longer have to complete endless forms; they just show their card and pay a small fee at the time of each visit. Most of the cost is paid by the insurer directly to the "provider" at contracted rates.

The industry is now beginning to apply its methods to Medicare and Medicaid patients in trial programs sponsored by the government. They feel that they will be able to improve the care of poor people previously underserved, just as they feel they have improved it for the general population.

Managed care contends that it has succeeded very well in controlling costs, reducing unnecessary and useless medical care, bringing accountability and measurement to a previously uncontrolled hodgepodge system, helping patients get coordinated care, and increasing preventive care. They feel that the competition and the financial incentives that are inherent in the new system will lead to continued improvement and that refinement of their methods will reduce any problems that have arisen from the strain of such a radical transformation in so short a time.

Is this rosy picture correct? Has managed care achieved the unthinkable—cheaper, better health care and high profits for the insurers? I wish that it were true, but I believe that it is not. I also believe that there are many reasons why managed *cannot* succeed, even if it is performed to the best degree possible, and that there are many reasons why it cannot achieve its lofty ideals.

In the following chapters we will explore why I believe this, where the problems might be, what the issues that must be considered are, and what might be better alternatives to this system of health care that so dominates the scene today.

1

Introduction

The good physician knows his patients through and through, and his knowledge is bought dearly. Time, sympathy, and understanding must be lavishly dispensed, but the reward is to be found in that personal bond which forms the greatest satisfaction of the practice of medicine. One of the essential qualities of the clinician is interest in humanity, for the secret of the care of the patient is in caring for the patient.

—Francis Weld Peabody, M.D.
Lecture to Harvard medical students, 1927

I run a $300-million-dollar business. You must think of patients as revenue flow. Greed and self-interest are the only incentives that matter in motivating physicians.

—Rationale of managed care as expressed to the author by a physician in charge of a large, predominantly managed care, hospital-sponsored clinic, 1997

We are all patients at some time, but today our lives and our health are at risk from the very system from which we would seek help. The health and life of every one of us has been put in danger for the simple advancement of someone else's financial profit. Corporate America has taken control of health care in this country and has forced the transformation of the practice of medicine from a noble profession to a mere money-driven business.

The health and well-being of patients were once the sacred trust of a profession grounded on the highest ethical principles that have endured over more than two thousand years. *In less than forty years, that tradition of nearly two millennia has been dangerously eroded.*

You the patient have become a commodity. Do you want to be revenue flow for some distant number cruncher for whom you are only a faceless unit? This change has been accomplished by a tactic that has allowed demagogues to conquer throughout history, namely, The Big Lie. The revolution succeeded on the promise to replace a falsely accused system with a supposedly better one that would deliver high-quality care at a low price. But promising everything for nothing is little more than the snake oil salesman coming back to haunt us. If you believe that cutting the heart out of the health care delivery system and denying critical benefits with very little, if any, savings is a good deal, then I have a bridge in Brooklyn I would like to sell you. **I will attempt in this book to show how we as a nation can have *good* care or *low-cost* care, but we cannot have *low-cost good care.***

In business, one uses all means possible, within basic ethical and legal limits, to achieve bottom-line results. One might feel that that is just what medicine needs—the business types who will eliminate waste, increase efficiency, and lower costs. The problem is that medicine is unlike any other service. Curing disease, preventing illness, maintaining fitness, and solving complex social and emotional problems are not on par with selling groceries or computers. People are not contracts, numbers, and inventory. Doctors are not "providers"—they are physicians and healers.

Government control might seem the best solution to some. Make no mistake, government is great for large-scale projects, for enforcing basic rights and standards, and for guaranteeing equal access to all. But it has no place in the personal choices and decisions of individuals.

The intrusion of business and government into individuals' health care has caused severe damage in many ways and has endangered the very heart and soul of medicine, namely the relationship between a doctor and his or her patient.

The doctor-patient relationship is the essence of medicine. It is *the* critical tool in the care of patients, in finding and treating disease, in preventing disease, and in helping patients maintain health and vigor. It is this, the most powerful weapon in the war against disease, that is most threatened today.

Doctor and patient share a unique relationship. When you first consult a doctor, he or she is a stranger. Yet you share your most intimate secrets with this stranger and allow yourself to be touched and probed in ways you would allow few others to do. The doctor must be both caring and objective, operating at peak performance at all times, with little room for error.

Good medical care takes time. It takes freedom from other parties intruding on your privacy and your right to decide your own care. It means that your doctor works only for you and does not have to answer to an insurance provider or some government bureaucrat. It means you are the physician's only employer at that moment, so there is no question of divided loyalty. It means absolute trust, for you are putting in the doctor's hands all that is most precious to you.

Today, government, business people, lawyers, and well-intentioned bureaucrats gain access to your most private records, steal the time you should have with your doctor, and increasingly restrict your choices and decisions. Business and government are mounting a massive assault on the doctor-patient relationship and the damage will be complete and irreparable if we do not act soon.

Virtually all discussion on health care today is about cost, with perfunctory attention paid to "quality." I believe we must redirect the debate to the care that patients actually receive in their doctors' offices. What was said of the dying salesmen, Willy Loman, can be said equally truly for the steady destruction of quality and ethics in health care: "Attention must be paid!"[1]

* * *

The debate on health care has been conducted among politicians, businesspeople, academics, lawyers, economists, and a limited number of executives from large physician organizations. Real doctors, the ones busy caring for patients every day, and the patients themselves have been excluded or ignored. This book speaks for all of us—everyone who is or will be a patient—and for the practicing physicians and nurses who devote their lives to providing that care.

President Clinton's much-maligned health care initiative gathered panels of over five hundred alleged experts, but not a single practicing physician or any ordinary people. Around that time, news anchor Ted Koppel hosted a two-hour town meeting on TV. Dozens of people spoke, but no practicing physicians were heard. This exclusion has been the case in virtually every forum and continues to this day. Recently, a four-day conference on managed care was held that did not include a single patient or a single practicing physician. When I asked the organizer about this, she said that I was wrong, that some of the physician speakers saw a few patients on the side.

Medicine is not seeing a few patients on the side! The *true* practice of medicine is sitting by the bedside of a dying patient in her home. Not all diseases can be cured, and when all treatments have been exhausted, there is nothing further for the doctor to do, but everything to give by just being there. It is talking every day to a seemingly comatose patient who everyone else assumes is completely unaware. When that patient finally improves after weeks in an intensive care unit and tells you that your words were the only things that kept him sane and gave him a will to keep living, you have given something no bureaucrat can measure.

Practicing medicine means coming to know your patient so well that for the first time in forty years he can share a secret that has scarred his life only because it was too painful to tell anyone. Once spoken, the patient then learns that what seemed so terrible to him as a child can be dealt with and he can finally begin to mend his life and find happiness. Practicing medicine means listening to all the foolish little fears that are overwhelming until exposed to the reassurance of a caring doctor who understands that there are no foolish fears, only concerns to be relieved. It means going beyond the obvious and helping patients with problems they did not even realize they had. It means being there not just for the patient but for the family as well. It means knowing about the whole social and economic environment in which the patient lives, since no problems exist in a vacuum. It means taking time to *listen* to the patient. It means being someone the patient can trust.

* * *

I am a practicing physician. This book is the culmination of over thirty years' experience across the entire range of medicine. I have trained and taught in many of the finest medical schools in the country and have practiced in nearly every kind of medical setting. Each patient I see adds something new to my daily experience and my own research on patient education, quality of patient care, and patient advocacy. Most research examines large groups in controlled conditions, but the doctor-patient relationship is not susceptible to traditional research methods. It is too personal, too individual to be categorized statistically.

What I have done instead is to observe and practice medicine in a very disparate set of conditions and populations, developing techniques and observations about the doctor-patient relationship that can then be disseminated more broadly. There has been inadequate attention paid to this crucial interaction even though it has been the heart of medical care since the time of Hippocrates, the great champion of the profession of healing.

* * *

I love medicine, as my father did before me, but I despise what it is becoming. I believe there are better ways to handle the cost of medical care than by destroying the very heart of caring medical practice. Certainly we must spend our money wisely, but we need not give up our souls to do so. In the rush to profit from the new managed care system, patient needs are being sacrificed to greed. We are all patients at one time or another and we all have a critical stake in the future of health care. What I hope to contribute to the debate is twofold: a sense of the real effects as felt directly by you and me and every patient and practicing physician, and a perspective on the debate from a real person's—a real doctor's—point of view, not that of a politician, theorizer, or businessperson.

Medicine has undergone several major transformations. Hippocrates, the ancient Greek physician, established the first ethical foundations of medicine, but otherwise superstition and ignorance ruled until the scientific method we know today emerged in the seventeenth century. As the scientific approach proved successful, its dominance accelerated with Louis Pasteur and his contemporaries in the nineteenth century and has grown exponentially since.

Though research was developing new tools and knowledge, the delivery of medical care was a poorly trained trade that harmed as much as it helped. At the turn of the twentieth century, Sir William Osler, Abraham Flexner, and others established high standards of teaching, patient care, and research and in the process created the modern medical school. The practice of medicine was transformed from a trade to a high profession and doctors began to heal and help far more effectively.

Sanitation, public health methods, immunization, and antibiotics eliminated epidemics and prevented or cured many infectious diseases, allowing more people to live long enough to develop chronic diseases, which have been the predominant focus since then. As medicine became more effective, doctors rose in the public's esteem.

In the 1960s, medicine changed again when the public assistance program known as Medicare brought the intrusive arm of government into medical care. This solved some of the problems of the elderly poor, by making basic health care affordable to those who previously could not afford it, but the seeds of destruction of the doctor-patient relationship were planted.

We are now in the midst of a new, equally significant change: the preemption of the control of medicine by businesspersons in the name of "managed care." Medicine has been transformed once again, this time from a profession to a business. The driving force of medicine has degenerated from the goal of giving patients the best care possible to that of reducing inflation of health care costs, saving money for corporations, and earning the greatest profit for the executives and stockholders of managed care companies.

Physicians were once the most respected members of society in every survey. Today, their standing is plummeting as these changes increasingly damage the relationship that brought a special bond between doctors and the people they serve.

We will examine the history of how medicine has reached its current state, what the problems have been, and how managed care and governmental intervention have not only *not* solved most of the problems, but have actually created far more serious ones. And we will explore how medicine can evolve into a system that serves everyone fairly.

Managed care as we know it now will likely decline and fade away. The companies that are now flourishing will do so only as long as they can attract young, healthy customers who pay premiums but don't use the services extensively, and so long as cost controls can be imposed without significant opposition. As their share of the medical care market currently continues to expand, two forces are combining to destroy their business: They are finding themselves having to pay for expensive sick and elderly patients who are heavy users of health care services, while their cost controls are being eroded by the inevitable backlash against their predatory business practices.* As premiums increase, corporations that must provide health care insurance to attract qualified employees will look elsewhere for new answers to providing that care at a lower cost.

---

*Beginning in 1997 and accelerating throughout the spring and summer of 1998, polls showed that public feeling toward managed care had turned sharply negative. Politicians rushed to assuage this dissatisfaction with an avalanche of state and federal laws and proposals to regulate managed care and reverse perceived abuses. The more that managed care is limited in its cost-cutting methods, the higher premiums will rise and the more the companies will attempt to restrict benefits to maintain profits.

The failure of managed care will leave a new void, to be filled by the next opportunistic plan, just as managed care filled the void left by the failure of President Clinton's health care reform plan.

Left to the natural flow of economic forces, I believe that the next step will be a combination of an expansion of a Medicare-type national health insurance, funded by direct premiums rather than payroll deductions, and the emergence of physician-operated managed care (called POSs). The other possibility would be a single national government health plan in which all physicians will be required to be employees of the system.

Unfortunately, any federal plan would be an enormous drain on government resources and would magnify the detrimental effects of bureaucracy to a degree that would make today's layer of departments and agencies seem small by comparison. Physician-run managed care will still be managed care, with all its attendant difficulties.

What *should* happen is that we should return to the roots of medicine: individual doctors, functioning freely, providing direct care to the people of the community in which they live, without interference. That system could have been preserved, with minimal modifications that would have countered unnecessary price inflation. The best control on cost and waste is the consumer who must spend his or her own funds. Had the system been changed so that patients always had to pay a part of the bill, they would choose carefully, and as long as the cost was not so high as to make care unaffordable, costs would have been reasonably contained.

Sadly, we can probably never return to that seemingly idyllic way of life, any more than Pandora could return the spirits of jaded knowledge and sin to the box that should have been their eternal trap. However, I believe that we can design a new health care system that will preserve the best of the old ways while meeting the needs of an America entering a new millennium. We will discuss this in the last chapter of this book.

Another problem is that we have too many uninsured or underinsured people, a situation that could only be described as a national disgrace. They are predominantly middle-class working families who are above Medicaid income levels and therefore don't qualify for coverage but whose employers do not pay for insurance. Some are uninsured only briefly, others choose to go without coverage, but many are suffering for reasons beyond their control. This last, large group, are those who cannot afford their own insurance and who are unemployed or work for companies that do not offer health insurance.

Every citizen should have access to a basic, satisfactory level of health care. Even if equity and compassion are not considered, it is an issue for everyone because the uninsured population actually increases health care costs.

How to solve the dilemma of providing affordable decent health care to everyone while preserving the doctor-patient relationship, the rights of doctors and patients, and the invaluable traditions of medicine will be the primary focus of this book. To do so, we must first explore what good medicine is and how it is being endangered.

NOTE

1. Arthur Miller, *Death of a Salesman* (New York: Viking Press, 1949), p. 56.

2

The Good Doctor: What Medical Care Should Be

I will follow that method of treatment which, according to my ability and judgment, I consider for the benefit of my patients, and abstain from whatever is deleterious and mischievous. I will give no deadly medicine to anyone if asked, nor suggest any such counsel.

With purity and Holiness I will pass my life and practice my art. Into whatever houses I enter I will go into them for the benefit of the sick and will abstain from every voluntary act of mischief and corruption.

Whatever, in connection with my professional practice, or not in connection with it, I may see or hear in the lives of men which ought not to be spoken abroad I will not divulge, as reckoning that all such should be kept secret.

While I keep this oath unviolated may it be granted to me to enjoy life and the practice of the art, respected by all men at all times, but should I trespass and violate this oath, may the reverse be my lot.

—Excerpts from the Oath of Hippocrates, approximately 400 B.C.E.
(Many versions exist, but the basics are the same
and are sworn to by medical students before
they are awarded their medical degrees at graduation.)

The principles of professionalism embodied in the Oath of Hippocrates have endured for over two thousand years. Yet it has taken less than forty years to nearly destroy the traditions of two millennia. Medicine's long history of strict professionalism and high integrity has been badly eroded. We have come far afield from the caring physician of Francis Weld Peabody, quoted at the beginning of this book, to today's physician executives who crunch numbers.

The primary responsibility of a business is to the bottom line—the profitability and continued existence of the business—and to the shareholders. Income is everything and often with adherence only to a narrow interpretation of the law and ethics.

I once asked a friend, a decent and responsible executive of a small chemical company, if he would protect his workers from danger if he knew his factory was exposing them to dangerous fumes. He said he would be concerned about the cost but would feel obligated to act. I then asked him if he did anything to protect them *in case* there were as yet *unrecognized* dangers to his employees. He said he would not because his first responsibility was to his shareholders and that he could not justify the expense. How many of his employees may have suffered medical illness over the years from hazards for which he never bothered to take precautions?

This executive was not a bad person and I am sure many other executives would give the same answer. On the other hand, if they felt that unrecognized hazards might pose undue future *financial* risks, they would take preventive action to prevent future *monetary* losses.

A free market advocate would then say that that is the beauty of capitalism, that good things get done for sound economic reasons, not theoretical philosophizing. Unfortunately, it often does not work out that way. When it fails in business, money and jobs are lost, both of which can be remedied. When health is lost, it is far more often irretrievable and the consequences far greater.

Medicine must take a different approach. Preserving health and preventing even unlikely consequences always takes priority over cash flow and cost. Obviously, there is some point at which the risk and the cost cross lines and thus there are limits. Where to draw the line between cost and risk is an underlying and essential question in the entire health care debate. We will discuss this critical question in the last chapter.

Medicine must be a profession, not a business, which means that the primary standard is the best care that can be provided to the patient, with the highest level of trustworthiness, skill, and respect for ethics. Income must always be secondary to maintaining the highest standards.

The Talmud, one of the most important books of laws and reasoning of Judaism, says, in effect, that physicians providing medical care are giving a mitzvah—a gift in honor of God for which no reward should be expected. The Talmud then says that while physicians should not be paid for their services, they must live and support their families, so they should be compensated for the income they forgo by choosing to be a doctor instead of some other job.

While the end result is the same—the doctor gets paid and earns a living—the distinction is important because it says that medicine is not mere commerce, but a calling to do good for others.

Doctors have a covenant with their patients, not a contract.*

In this chapter, we shall examine what medicine should be and what constitutes quality care, all of which is currently in great jeopardy.

* * *

What should you reasonably expect from your doctor? (Some aspects of what follows apply more to internal medicine than to other specialties, but the basic principles are the same for all. Obviously, a radiologist reading an X-ray has different needs than an internist seeing a patient; a surgeon's use of time is different from that of a psychiatrist.)

CONFIDENTIALITY

The right to be let alone is the most comprehensive of rights and the right most valued in civilized man.

—Supreme Court Justice Louis Brandeis

Confidentiality is the obligation to keep *private* all that is said and transpires between doctor and patient related to the patient's care and medical information. It is a legal, ethical, and moral obligation, with few exceptions.

The information the patient gives the doctor is the most important diagnostic tool there is. Understanding a medical problem begins first

*While, legally, covenants and contracts are both written documents to be signed and sealed, with little distinction, in common use and in religion covenant has a far different implication. In the history of medicine and in discussions of medical ethics, covenant has meant the unspoken but inherent promise to do the best possible to beneift the patient. When a patient consults a physician, there is no written contract between them that states that the physician will treat the patient according to the highest standards and traditions of medicine, but every patient *expects* that and by definition every *good* physician promises that. Good physicians answer to a higher calling than the written word. Beneficence is the highest aspiration of medicine and simply means doing good. Sir William Osler, the great professor of medicine, said "The profession of medicine is distinguished from all others by its singular beneficence." The covenant of medicine is the promise of beneficence.

and foremost with the patient's medical history, with what the patient *says*. Information you withhold from your doctor may endanger your health or even your life. Most people will understandably be very reluctant to reveal things about themselves if they feel other people might have access to the information without their knowledge or permission. However, a patient may not realize that his or her privacy is at risk. For example, many people do not read or comprehend the life and health insurance contracts they sign. Few notice the obscure release clause that permits the insurance company total access to patient records.

When patients apply for life insurance they are required to release their medical records for review. I often get requests from insurance companies to photocopy an entire patient record and to send it to them. I always refuse and instead send a summary that includes only the minimal information needed by the underwriting department. It takes me much longer, but I do not believe that patients should have to reveal the intimate details of their lives to some distant stranger and have their records at the mercy and control of insurers just to see if they qualify for a product being sold for profit.

Our minds are the one thing over which we—and only we—have complete control. There are things that we choose to keep private for many reasons, sometimes even from our dearest loved ones. It is our choice alone, but there are times when we need to confide in a doctor for help and advice. That is possible only with the confidence that it will be completely private.

The exceptions to confidentiality are few and extremely limited. They include a legal subpoena (but even this has restrictions as to specific relevant information) and certain public health laws (that vary from state to state) that are essential to limit the spread of highly contagious diseases or other dangerous public health conditions. If, for example, another doctor is brought in as part of your care, such as a consultant, a doctor who covers for your doctor while he is sick or on vacation or unable to attend to your needs, or someone doing a test or procedure, he or she needs to know enough to carry out his or her function. The referring doctor should discuss only what is essential.

Another exception might arise in an emergency where immediate decisions are needed to save a life or prevent serious injury. Similarly, where someone is unconscious or unable to handle his or her affairs and there is no pre-existing health directive, the doctor may have to turn to the most reasonable surrogate for the patient.

You, of course, can release your information to whomever you wish. Your doctor, however, is far more restricted regarding to whom he can divulge information.

Many threats to your medical privacy already exist and, as we will see, it can get much worse.

WHOM DOES YOUR DOCTOR SERVE?

The only right answer to the above question is *you*, the patient. Originally, it was that simple. The patient, with the doctor's assistance, decided what the best course of treatment would be. No one else was involved in the decision, with few exceptions. The doctor's only employer, in effect, was the patient. The only standards to be met were the patient's and, of course, the highest standards of informed and ethical medical practice. It was not an idyllic time and there were other sorts of problems, but the freedom from outside intervention was a major advantage.

Then it began to change, until doctors today are, in effect, most often employed by insurance companies and the government. The patient who thinks he or she has consulted a doctor has actually become the customer of either a large, usually profit-driven entity or the government, without even realizing it.

Doctors now answer to many bosses. Medicine *should* be practiced as a doctor and a patient sitting down together for the sole purpose of helping the patient. Instead, present in the room with them today, unseen but often pulling the strings, are an insurance clerk, a lawyer, and a government bureaucrat.

The insurance company or the government pays the bills, sets the rules, and makes the final decisions as to treatment by determining what procedures are covered by medical plans. Lawyers, government bureaucrats, and others look over the doctor's shoulder, second-guessing all decisions. The doctor knows that if these many bosses are not pleased, severe financial repercussions can occur, not to mention the legal and even psychological damage.

Each patient is unique. The diseases may be the same, but the picture is different for each patient. You can make rules that apply to three cases of breast cancer, but you cannot make rules that apply properly to three women with breast cancer, for they are three entirely different situations. The disease may be the same in each but the unique characteristics of each person make every case different. Doctors take care of people; companies and governments take care of diseases. *You* want to be taken care of by a doctor.

TIME

Time is the most valuable thing a man can spend.

—Theophrastus

Do not squander time, for that is the stuff life is made of.

—Benjamin Franklin

Time stays long enough for anyone who will use it.

—Leonardo da Vinci

Time is the most precious commodity for us all—it cannot be made, changed, or stopped, and there is a strictly limited supply for each of us. Time is essential to good medical care. Consider what is involved in a medical visit:

- The greeting: Patients are often anxious seeing a doctor. The first step is to put the patient at ease and help him or her feel comfortable. If new to the doctor, some conversation to get to know the patient is essential. Even idle conversation or discussions about the news, the patient's family, work, interests, and the like are very informative because personality and background will emerge from that much more than from formal questions.
- Taking the history: The doctor listens as the patient describes, in his or her own words, the symptoms that have prompted the visit. How the problem developed, associated symptoms and problems, whether there is any past history applicable to the current problem, what actions the patient may have taken already, and what the patient seeks to accomplish need to be discussed. With new patients, it is vital to establish a baseline with a thorough and complete general history.

  Taking a history is a true skill and art. Probing the complete background, past history, lifestyle, and personal history of someone you have just met is no easy task. When done properly, patients will feel comfortable and communicate everything.

  An experienced doctor may know you better in a short while

than most of your friends will no matter how long they have known you. A skilled doctor can read people very quickly, learning about a patient from body language and appearance as well as from what is being said.

- The exam: Performing a physical exam is another important skill, one that is gradually dying out as medical students learn technology at the expense of direct examination. A professor in medical school once spent four hours teaching me physical examination, and we only got down to the neck! A physical exam can be done efficiently in a reasonable time, though it is important not to be tempted to cut corners.
- Tests: These are sometimes done by assistants, but there are some that require the doctor's participation. In either case, the doctor must first explain what the tests are, why they are needed, and any discomforts or risks entailed.
- Assessment and counseling: The doctor explains to the patient the initial impression of the problem and what is advised to be done about it.

The first session may be just preliminary, but once more test results are available, the doctor has much to communicate to the patient. This communication must be in terms the patient can understand. Jargon is useful, precise shorthand for communicating with colleagues, but it is gibberish to anyone not in medicine, so the doctor must be careful to speak in understandable terms. It is even more than just the language. The doctor must tailor his or her approach to the style, background, educational level, and beliefs of the patient.

Reading the above, it is obvious that all this takes a fair amount of time. There was a fad in the 1980s to talk about working parents' "quality time" with their children, as if a limited time doing something special was as good as spending a lot of time with the child. (The comic strip "Doonesbury," by Gary Trudeau, did a strip in which a "parenting expert" says that quality time is coming home and spending a good fifteen minutes with your child meeting his needs. He is asked what if the child's needs are more time with the parent and he answers that they are not talking about the *problem* child.) In truth, quality time with children is spending time with them, no matter what you do. The *more* time you spend the better. (I told my son once when he was four that I loved being with him even if all we did was read the telephone book. Ever since, even years later, he still looks at me occasionally with a smile and asks if I want to read the telephone book with him. If my daughter is reading, I will quietly come and sit next to her. She is soon cuddled next to me without missing a word. My being there is what counts.) There may be good or inescapable reasons to be away from your children and to make the most of the time when you are with them, but make no mistake, quantity counts.

Quantity of time spent is equally important in patient care.

For a doctor, time is precious because income is earned only while the physician is actually working and there are enormous calls and drains on that very limited resource. The very fact that a doctor spends a generous amount of that time with a patient is in itself a very important message to the patient that he or she matters and that the doctor cares. When people remember what they like about popular politicians, the most nearly universal remark I have heard (most recently in a remembrance of President Kennedy) is to the effect that when the politician talked with them it seemed as if the politician felt that no one else in the world mattered at that moment. You want to have that feeling about your doctor, because the problem you have come for is vitally important to you.

All that I just described in the doctor-patient encounter takes a great deal of *time* if it is to be done effectively. Anything that reduces that time reduces the quality and effectiveness of health care. As we will see, managed care and government steal time that should be spent on your care.

LISTENING

Hearing is one of the body's five senses. But listening is an art.

—Frank Tyger

It is not enough just to *hear*—you have truly to listen to what is being said. Listening is a skill that must be learned, like any other skill. Listening comes in many forms. Many times patients ask me about some innocent little bump that is obviously nothing. If I were just to say it is nothing, few people would be reassured. What I almost always say instead is, "First of all, it is not a cancer. . . ." I usually don't get to finish the sentence because the patient has heard what he wanted to hear, gives a big sigh of relief, and needs nothing else. Thus listening means hearing what is unsaid as well as what is spoken.

Some patients come with many minor complaints. A good cost-effectiveness manager would shun such visits as a waste of the doctor's valuable time, and a drain on resources. Yet, those complaints are extremely important to that person. Furthermore, for some patients the many little complaints are not the problem, but are just a screen for some far more serious problem, physical or emotional, which the patient finds too painful to voice. With patience, time, and gentle questioning, the physician can help the patient to talk about the real problem.

Patients must also listen well or they will miss the information for which they came to the doctor in the first place. Most of us have short attention spans. We listen to the first few words and assume the rest. Many people are so anxious to get their thoughts out that they are beginning the next question before you have finished answering the first. Why ask a question if you do not listen to the answer?

Some patients ask the same question repeatedly hoping that if they ask it often enough the answer will change to what they want to hear. What they really want is validation of their hopes and beliefs.

I watch patients carefully to see if they are absorbing what I am saying or if they have not really accepted it. The information is so important to their health that I keep coming back to it until I am sure they have it.

Many years ago, before the Sperry-Rand Corporation was swallowed up in mergers and name changes, the then chairman of the board spent considerable corporate funds on an ad campaign that consisted solely of a series of essays on the lost art of listening. When interviewed, he said he was just so frustrated that no one listened to any one else anymore that he wanted to do what he could to change that. Few people listened to him, of course.

INDIVIDUALITY

The doctor needs to know the individual with basic, expert, and specialized understanding if he is to work with success. He sees men of all ages from childhood to senility. He is present at birth and at death. He observes man in his confidence of full health and in his fear of sickness. He observes him near the noon of day when courage is at its height, and in the small hours of the morning when it so often ebbs away. Not only must he understand the individual, but he must understand him in many of these variations from the norm.

—Sir James Calvert Spence, *The Purpose and Practice of Medicine*

Each of us is unique. It is more likely to find two snowflakes that are identical than to find two people who are the same. Even identical twins have their differences.

Doctors see the same problems every day. Internists will see many patients with hypertension (high blood pressure), cardiologists will see many patients with chest pains, and rheumatologists will see lots of painful joints. Just treating the same complaints every day could be very boring.

I never get bored because I do not treat diseases, I treat people who have diseases. People are not boring. Every patient becomes a challenge if you see each as the unique person he or she is. You are not a runny nose, an atherosclerotic heart, or a breast cancer. You are a living being with a life and feelings and needs who may have a disorder in one part of your system. Each disease, from the lowly common cold to the most aggressive cancer, is different in each person. We teach medical students that the diseases do not read the textbooks. Doctors must look beyond the standard presentation of a condition or they will miss many cases.

Attitude and state of mind have extraordinary effects on the perception of health. I once saw two patients during the same six-month period. As dress inspectors, they worked side by side in a dress warehouse. All day long, bending and straightening, they examined long dresses from top to bottom for flaws or bad seams. One woman's complaint was that she had a bad neck and that it was too painful for her to work. Every test and exam showed no objective evidence of a physical cause for her pain. Nevertheless, she persisted and went out on permanent long-term disability.

The other woman continued to work, despite the same backbreaking job and a two-hour commute one way, until two weeks before she died of the widespread breast cancer that had spread throughout her bones the entire time. She and I both knew what she had all along and she was receiving treatment, but she never complained and she declined all of my suggestions for reduced hours.

What kept one woman at work despite the severe pain of advanced cancer while another stayed at home with a minor complaint?

Another patient came to my office with very painful rheumatoid arthritis. She was in her late sixties and had just lost her husband. As she and her daughter sat with me, I could tell she was very depressed; she would not speak or even look at me. We tried different medications to relieve her pain and swelling but nothing worked and eventually she was hospitalized.

As I tended to make hospital rounds very late, I was able to see her without her family around and she began to talk to me. I spent time chatting with her in her room, which she shared with three other patients. One night I came particularly late, near midnight. She was the only one awake, sitting cross-legged on her bed. I asked why she wasn't asleep. She was reluctant to tell me; she said I would think she was crazy. I gently encouraged her to go on.

Finally, she said that she kept seeing her dead husband sitting at her bedside accusing her of being a bad wife. They had been married many decades and he had grown bitter and irritable during his long terminal illness and had been very hard on her. She admitted, although she was ashamed to say it, that she had grown to hate him, and she felt a wife should never hate her husband. She felt guilty that she had been in another room when he collapsed and died.

In truth, of course, she had been a wonderful wife, caring for him all those years despite his being so hard on her. I told her that, and that she was entitled to resent being so verbally abused. I also pointed out that she did not really hate him but rather the disease he suffered from and what it had turned him into at the end.

She brightened for the first time and asked me if I was sure it was all right. I again reassured her and she went to sleep immediately. I saw her the next morning and she was smiling and cheerful, ready to go home. Her joints were still swollen and red but now she said she hardly felt the pain. Her arthritis had not changed, but her attitude and perception had.

The mind is very powerful. People are not bodies with brains on top, they are complex beings in which body, mind, and personality constantly interact. The good physician must listen to all three, must know the beliefs and environment that shape the person, and must see him or her as a whole person, not simply a collection of organs.

BEYOND THE OFFICE

As the preceding examples show, our health is not just a physical matter, but a synthesis of mind, body, and emotion. Even that is only part of someone's life, for none of us lives in a vacuum. Our financial status, our family life and social contacts, our work or lack of it, our home and environment—all play their separate critical roles in our health and well-being and in whatever goes wrong. I still make house calls whenever I can, though it is becoming increasingly difficult because I learn a tremendous amount about patients from seeing them at home in their own environment.

In the early years of medical discovery, science seemed to vanquish the then major cause of disease, infections (which have shown themselves to be no easy conquest after all). As these successes allowed people to live long enough to develop chronic diseases, science discovered that "cure" was not as easy as it looked. We then rediscovered what ancient and (allegedly) primitive people have long known: that it is impossible to separate mind, body, and environment in understanding life and its disorders. These concepts are not philosophy; they are practical and concrete necessities in patient care. We have discussed the interactions of mind, body, and emotion, but equally important is the environment in which the patient lives.

Charles Longino and Eric Cassel have written extensively on these issues.[1] They give a hypothetical example to illustrate, which I will summarize:

A seventy-eight-year-old man who was found unconscious in his apartment is brought to the emergency room. He is found to have pneumonia and chronic arthritis of one knee. His pneumonia is cured and he is returned home, only to be readmitted soon after with an even worse pneumonia.

Had the disinterested house staff looked beyond what seemed like an obvious and uninteresting case, they would have discovered the whole story.

The man lived alone in a fifth-floor walk-up. He had recently lost his wife. He was depressed, stopped seeing anyone, became more isolated and depressed and lost his appetite, but in any case did not go out for groceries because his knee hurt too much. This led to malnutrition, which weakened his immune system, which allowed him to develop pneumonia.

He was readmitted because on returning home he became more depressed, turned to alcohol, which caused him to vomit, some of which went into his lungs, causing a more serious pneumonia.

The senior doctor advised the house staff that they could cure him and send him home but they could not keep him out of the hospital unless they looked at the whole picture and found a way for the man to get help at home and companionship to help him through his period of grief and mourning.

Spending time to find out all about your patient is a critical element in treating patients properly.

SKILLS, KNOWLEDGE, CAREFULNESS, AND THOROUGHNESS

As important as all the above is, it is just as important that the doctor knows what he or she is doing! The doctor must know medicine; be well trained to begin with; and, since medicine is changing, expanding and improving daily, must keep up to date. Doctors must never stop learning, or, as is alleged of sharks if they stop swimming, they will drown.

It is impossible for any of us doctors to know all of medicine any more, even in our own field. Fortunately, we do not have to memorize every fact. A medical student is exposed to an estimated 13,000 new words in the first year alone, which is more than most people's entire vocabulary. No one can remember it all. What we ***must know*** is how to think and diagnose, where and how to find information, what is available for diagnosis and treatment and how to apply it. The system that has stood us in good stead for centuries is where one physician cares for the patient and calls in consulting specialists to assist where a specific skill or knowledge is needed. If the patient just sees different specialists, then his organs are cared for but the patient is not. As in the old saying, it is as if the operation were a success but the patient died.

I receive over thirty journals a month. I do not read everything in them, but I make sure I have a good overview of what I do not read. I make every consultation a learning experience. I look up everything I have the slightest doubt about. It is a continual struggle.

There are doctors who seem to know every fact, but nevertheless, they are not always very good doctors. It takes more than facts. Of equal importance is recognizing what you don't know. I tell patients that three of the most important words in medicine are "I don't know." Doing the wrong thing is as bad as doing nothing. If you know that there is something you do not know, then you can find out what to do. But if you think you know it all, you might harm someone without realizing you are overextending your skills.

It is still not enough just to have knowledge and skill. You must be driven to be careful and thorough. Doctors can never afford to let their guard down. Medicine is exhausting not just because of the long hours, but also because you must be at peak energy at all times that you are seeing patients. One sloppy moment can mean harm to someone.

None of us is perfect and we will all make mistakes no matter how hard we try to be careful and alert, but the harder we try, the closer we will come to freedom from error. When I see a patient, I can usually tell what's wrong within the first few minutes. I do not stop with my first impression, however; I always look further and sometimes things are not what they first seemed. Every patient is an individual and we must be careful and thorough at all times. I approach every patient encounter on edge. If I ever lose that, if I become complacent, I will stop seeing patients.

This thoroughness is essential to good care. Doctors do many things that are low-yield because the stakes are so high. For example, there are various maneuvers on a physical exam that seldom reveal anything for the extra effort they require. When I begin to wonder whether I really need to keep doing that, it pays off on the next patient. There is no substitute for being thorough and complete with each patient, within, reason of course.

OBJECTIVITY

When speaking with your family and friends and even with strangers, there is always an interaction beyond words. We all carry our own feelings, beliefs, style, fears, and history with that person. The feedback you get from others is never a clear mirror—it is always colored by their interpretation. Yet, we need feedback all the time. You cannot tell me what is on your forehead nor I, mine, but we can tell each other or look in a mirror. We are always looking from the inside out at our problems and need others to provide the perspective of distance.

When we need objective feedback, uncolored by relationships, we turn to a professional. One of the skills doctors must learn is to be objective, to divorce their own feelings and judgments from their encounters with patients. You should feel free to express *anything* to a doctor without having to concern yourself with the doctor's judgment of you.

It may seem impossible, but good doctors can really listen objectively. Just as they handle bodily fluids and other usually unpleasant things without flinching, so can they handle unpleasant revelations from patients. Doctors do not lose their distaste for those fluids away from patient care and they certainly have their own opinions, but they do not (or should not) apply judgments to patients. The patient should never feel embarrassed and reluctant to share feelings and information.

Objectivity is essential to good practice, but it does not mean that the doctor cannot *care* about the patient. Caring for a patient without caring for the person is not medicine, it's just mechanics.

CARING

As I have made as clear as possible, caring is an essential part of good medical care. Economist Victor Fuchs, in his influential 1974 book, *Who Shall Live?* attempts to differentiate "caring" from "curing."[2] He begins with the oft quoted but erroneous assumption that most of what medicine does is not curative. It may have been truer in 1974 than today, but even then, the figures were exaggerated.

The claim is that 80 percent of visits to doctors are for purely functional problems, meaning that there is no physical basis for the symptoms that the patient came for, that they are instead secondary to stress, anxiety, fear, or other emotional causes. The further claim is that half of the remaining 20 percent cannot be helped at all, which would mean that doctors make a difference in only 10 percent of cases. This sounds wise and has been widely disseminated, but, unfortunately, is just plain wrong.

It is certainly true that emotional factors play an enormously important role, as is quite clear in the preceding sections. Some problems are completely functional, like the dress inspector with the sore neck; in others, like the two other women I described, the patients' emotional state greatly influences their physical state. It is also true that the common cold cures itself and that antibiotics are useless for viruses. In many conditions, treatments do not cure, they just relieve symptoms, which is nevertheless of great value.

However, in my experience, physical causes play a major role in at least 50 percent of visits. Medical intervention cures, controls, or significantly influences the outcome in *most* cases other than colds.

A doctor can make a major contribution to the patient's welfare whether the cause is functional or organic. Even the assurance that there is no physical cause can be of benefit, but only if the source of that reassurance is reliable.

If you experience chest pain, sweating, and weakness, you do not want some well-intentioned "caring" person to tell you not to worry, that it's all in your head, it's caused by stress. You want a real doctor to make sure that you are not experiencing a serious heart problem. If evaluation establishes that your heart is healthy, then you can work on coping with stress in better ways.

It is important to understand that in functional disease, the symptoms are as real as any organic symptoms. For example, dizziness can be due to physical or emotional causes, but the dizziness is real whichever cause it is from. A good doctor will use all the factors discussed previously to diagnose the problem correctly and to find the best solution, with the same degree of concern and effort whatever the cause.

The economic argument would be that it may require expensive and highly trained physicians to cure disease, but *anyone* can give "caring" by being warm and attentive and laying on soothing hands. Therefore, the obvious suggestion would be to use inexpensive caregivers for the "caring" and reserve the physicians just for "curing."

That may sound fine and logical to an economist sitting in his study, but it has nothing to do with medical reality. Treating patients that way is hazardous. Trying to separate caring and curing is like trying to separate Siamese twins who share a single heart; they are inextricably entwined. Caring without medical knowledge creates a high risk of missing the diagnosis, neglecting the organic aspects of the problem, overlooking the physical impact of the emotional stress, and consequently misdirecting efforts. Attempting to apply cures without caring is just blindly applying cookbook solutions and is contrary to all that makes a good physician.

Fuchs's book suggested hotlines and special centers, which he says will be "manned by volunteers and dedicated paraprofessionals expert in 'caring' by virtue of temperament and/or training. Such a service is probably most effective when provided by someone who cares by choice rather than by necessity." We have such people—they are called doctors.

Fuchs is a fine economist who has made valuable contributions and has raised important issues for discussion, but I believe he is way off base here. I am spending time on this because it is not just an idle theoretical discussion. Managed care is actively trying to put variants of this concept into practice today.

To reduce costs, cutbacks must be made somewhere. Always a tempting target are those pesky, expensive doctors. If we could just get rid of them and replace them with cheaper versions, wouldn't that be great? I suspect that most of the people making these suggestions would themselves see a doctor about their heart disease rather than an expert in caring or a lesser trained (less expensive) "paraprofessional."

Why not reserve the doctors for the serious problems needing cures and do everything else with the carer (we will have to have some name for them)? Well, suppose that you go to see a carer about your dizziness and palpitations. I suspect you would want your carer to be able to tell if you have stress or heart disease; hypochondria or an impending stroke; fatigue or serious anemia. Your carer may be stroking your hand reassuringly as your serious medical condition is spiraling toward disaster.

Well, then, the cost cutters would argue, we will just train our paraprofessionals to be alert for serious diseases that might need a real doctor. We have people trained like that—they are called doctors.

A good physician should *be* a physician. There is a real advantage to consulting someone who has successfully completed four years of college, four years of medical school, four years of postgraduate training, and who has sworn to the Hippocratic Oath.

THE PATIENT'S RIGHT TO SELF-DETERMINATION

Freedom is the last, best hope of Earth.
—Abraham Lincoln

The doctor-patient relationship has changed considerably in the last thirty years. Doctors used to be seen as all-knowing experts who told the patient what to do. Patients often saw themselves as needing to put themselves into the hands of an omniscient physician who would then fix them much as a mechanic fixes a car. Today, in most cases, the relationship has evolved to an equal partnership between doctor and patient with a mutual goal of solving the patient's problem and promoting health. Some patients still prefer just to be told what to do, taking comfort in the authority figure they create in their mind for reassurance, but they are probably the minority today. The doctor is now seen as an expert consultant to advise the patient in identifying the problems and the available choices for resolution. The decisions are the patient's, not the doctor's—after all, whose life is it anyway?

That was the concept of a play of similar title on Broadway over a decade ago, and later a movie. It crystallized the question by making the patient completely paralyzed from the neck down and at the complete mercy of the doctor who cared for him (or her, when Mary Tyler Moore played the part). The patient wanted to end his life, which held so little for him, but was completely dependent on the doctor to take that action.

This is a more complex question than that encountered in most situations, since a doctor's whole being is to relieve suffering and preserve life. How does the doctor resolve the conflict when the two objectives are mutually exclusive, when ending life may be the only way to relieve suffering? Hippocrates said, "I will give no deadly medicine to anyone if asked, nor suggest any such counsel." Most major religions would oppose it as well. Dr. Jack Kevorkian and others have forced a national debate on this very issue.

While the play poses an extreme instance, the principle of whose life is it is vitally important and universal. The answer in terms of law is a social decision, not a medical one. The answer in actual practice is that every case is individual and must be resolved by the conjunction of the patient's sovereignty over his or her life; the doctor's professional, moral, and ethical obligations and beliefs; the law; and good will.

It is equally important to realize how personal, how fundamental to all that we believe and stand for, how delicate are the patient's personal issues, whether about day-to-day mundane problems or matters of life and death. To have distant government bureaucrats or profit-driven agents of corporations inserted into these intensely personal decisions is outrageous and against all decency. Society must trust in the individual to determine his or her life, for that is the essence of democracy and freedom.

EDUCATION AND PREVENTION

Your doctor is your expert medical advisor. What do you want to learn? At the least you want to know about your current problem, the available options for treatment and the pros and cons of each. You want to be informed in terms you can understand. I feel strongly that every patient encounter, even when not as a general check-up, is an opportunity to look for problems the patient may not recognize and, equally important, to teach patients to be more fit and to prevent illness.

Age does not disable people, only disease does. One can be just as happy and productive at ninety as one can at twenty, albeit with some accommodation for the relatively minor changes of aging. Certainly, you are not the same at ninety as at twenty, but none of the changes is disabling or limiting of enjoyment of life. There are ninety-year-olds running marathons, sky diving, writing books, making beautiful music, and much more. The maximum human lifespan is at least 120 years and "old" is an obsolete term.

I spend a great deal of time with patients teaching them the best strategies to prevent disease, maintain fitness, and enjoy life. I believe that it is an essential part of all medical care for internists and other doctors who take care of the whole person. The critical point here is how much should a doctor do during a patient visit? Obviously, a visit for a serious acute illness is not the time for more general care. Also, specialties such as radiology and anesthesiology are intended for highly specialized and focused skills, not counseling on prevention.

Educating and informing *take time.* It is up to the patient to decide how much information he or she wants from the doctor, but the doctor should offer it and spend time on it if appropriate. Dr. David Seegal, one of the best professors I had in medical school and a renowned teacher and expert on medical education, taught that it is not enough to inform patients—you must *convince* them. What good is advice if it is not followed? Not all doctors agree; many feel their job is just to inform. Professor Seegal did not mean doctors should attempt to impose their view in some godlike manner. Instead, he meant that it was important to present the information so fully and relevantly that the patient can then sensibly decide what to do.

INFORMED CONSENT

> *The highest compact we can make with our fellow is: Let there be truth between us two forevermore.*
>
> —Ralph Waldo Emerson

"Informed consent" is a term lawyers use to describe good medical practice in ways that can yield profitable lawsuits. A good doctor will always tell a patient the risks and disadvantages of a treatment. The issue arises, how much detail is reasonable? How much should the doctor be able to anticipate?

The *1998 Physicians' Desk Reference* (PDR) is a 3,223-page book printed in minutely small type, three columns per page, published under the aegis of the pharmaceutical industry and the regulation of the FDA. It purports to include all information about medications requiring prescriptions. That is a lot of information.

Most of the drugs have very long lists of potential uses, side effects, adverse effects, risks, contraindications, drug interactions, and precautions. Drug companies list every single even slightly possible problem to prevent themselves from being accused of not warning of a risk. Thus, many of the risks listed are not realistic. Others are noted to occur in "less than 1 percent of cases."

What is informed consent? For a good doctor, it means telling the patient all of the *practical* potential problems and precautions. Legally, however, if the doctor omits one obscure adverse effect that the patient happens to be unlucky enough to suffer, the doctor may be held liable for lack of informed consent. One patient once sued claiming that the doctor had spent a lot of time advising but had not been convincing enough! (She did not win.) Thus, for legal protection, the doctor should force you to sit through the *entire* PDR write-up even if you do not want to hear it. Even if the doctor did that, there would be no witnesses to prove it so it would come down to whom the jury believed.

This is just one small example of that unseen lawyer sitting in on *your* visit to the doctor. Do you really want your doctor to treat you with one ear tuned to how it will sound in court, as the malpractice defense lawyers advise all doctors to do? Does this contribute to trust and the free flow of discussion between doctor and patient?

The correct meaning of "informed consent" is that the doctor must help the patient understand not just the risk of a treatment, but balance that against the risk of *not* taking the treatment. There is a small risk of an adverse effect from an antibiotic for a bacterial pneumonia, even a fatal risk, but there is a much greater risk of leaving the pneumonia untreated.

Likewise, there is balance between desired benefit and risk. A painful ankle is seldom fatal, but most people would not hesitate to take some Tylenol® or Advil® to feel better. Yet, both drugs can have serious, even fatal consequences if used incorrectly.

The best analogy is crossing the street. Even though you wait for the light to be in your favor and look both ways before proceeding, some crazy driver might come careening around the corner and run you down anyway. The alternative is never to cross the street, or, even safer, to hide under your bed hoping a meteorite does not hit your house. You might be safer but you would have no life.

Thus, we are taking risks all the time. Most of us do not give everyday risks a second thought, *until* we enter a doctor's office. Suddenly, perfectly reasonable people can seriously consider declining an essential treatment because they have heard something on television or read a long mandated list of extremely unlikely risks courtesy of our overly litigious society.

Patients deserve a *reasonable* risk-benefit analysis.

TRUST

A good doctor instills trust between him- or herself and the patient. No sane person will put his or her life in the hands of someone who was not trusted. Trust is fragile until there is a long enough experience to cement it. At times the simplest misspoken word or mistake can destroy it.

A patient who feels that the doctor owes allegiance to an employer other than the patient will begin to withhold trust and be reluctant to share personal information or to follow advice. If the doctor does not agree to a requested treatment or procedure because it is not right for the patient, the patient may not believe that is the reason and may assume it was to save money for the HMO.

Patients in managed care no longer feel confident that decisions are made for their benefit rather than for some cost-saving reason. Instead of teamwork between doctor and patient, it has become an adversarial contest.

The trust must be mutual. The doctor must feel secure that the patient will not abuse the relationship any more than the patient would expect of the doctor. Patients who make unreasonable demands, who repeatedly do not follow advice, or who misuse medications create difficulty for the doctor. An adverse outcome due to a patient's failure to follow carefully given instructions reflects on the doctor even if unjustified. At the least, it is very frustrating for the doctor.

Under managed care (and even under Medicaid and Medicare), doctors must continuously be afraid of complaints, which can be filed anonymously and falsely. Enough complaints, justified or not, and the doctor might lose a large contract and experience a major drop in income or face investigation by the government. The doctor is caught between the insurance carrier's desire that he do less and the threat of complaints from patients who feel they should have more. Even though the decision is not the doctor's, the doctor takes the heat.

In the absence of outside interference, an appreciative patient and a caring and thoughtful doctor can establish a relationship on a solid basis of trust and mutual respect. Sadly, this bond is being eroded, perhaps irretrievably, by the intrusion of government and business.

NOTES

1. Charles Longino, "Beyond the Body: An Emerging Medical Paradigm," *American Demographics* (December 1997): 14–19.

2. Victor Fuchs, *Who Shall Live?* (New York: Basic Books, 1974), pp. 64–67.

3

From Hippocrates to "Providers": How Healers and Caregivers Became Product Sellers

I know of no way of judging the future but by the past.
—Patrick Henry

In the history of medicine, what began as superstition and myth over 2500 years ago slowly evolved into elegantly logical science. Part of the story is told in a wonderful book called *Microbe Hunters,* by Paul de Kruif, published in 1928. It begins with a Dutch shopkeeper named Anton Leeuwenhoek, who lived from 1632 to 1723. He made microscopes more powerful and clearer than any ever before and used them, along with what today we call scientific method, to discover and learn about microbes.

The book goes on to describe the work of Louis Pasteur and other pioneers who paved the way that led to our success against infectious disease. Though de Kruif's history is oversimplified, he expressed the beauty, thrill, and challenge of science so well that many scientists have said it was the first spark that led them to their careers.

Studying medicine is extremely hard and dauntingly difficult, but what you learn is fascinating and when you finally finish medical school and begin to be out in the world again, it is hard to imagine *not* knowing what you have learned about being human.

My father graduated from The Johns Hopkins School of Medicine in 1933. Studying his books, microscope slides, and instruments from that era, I am amazed at how much was already known at that time and how rigorous was their science. William Osler and others at Hopkins had virtually invented the modern medical school, and many of the great professors were still there in 1933.

My father's fifty-eight year career spanned a period of remarkable change. He remembered the day the first anti-infectious agent, sulfonamide, was brought onto the wards at the Hopkins hospital in 1935. Before sulfonamide, all doctors could do was tenderly care for patients, give worthless serums and potions, and wait for the patient to survive or die. Then, suddenly, one day, they had only to give the patient the new medicine and, within hours, a doomed patient would be well on the way to recovery. Penicillin arrived soon after and went into wide use as the United States entered World War II, just in time to save many soldier and civilian lives (including the author as a toddler at the end of the war).

Wonderful new inventions, drugs, surgical techniques, and tests came at a rapid clip. These were literally miraculous developments and the new armamentarium boosted the status of American medicine to dizzying heights. Within that success would later sprout the seeds of trouble.

Contrast the life in America in 1850 with that of 1950. In 1850, most of the population lived on farms, in small towns, and in newly settled western regions. Most Americans had to be self-sufficient, and people generally determined their own way within small communities. There were few "experts" available and education was limited. Thus, doctors were seen as little more than tradespeople.

There were few hospitals and people were usually cared for at home by their family. Doctors were called sparingly. They could not do much, anyway, and too often they actually made the patient worse with harmful or misguided treatments. With so little to offer, doctors had limited prestige and authority, except in a few Eastern centers like New York, Philadelphia, and Boston.

There was no licensing, no standards, no Food and Drug Administration, and no national consensus, and anyone could sell worthless tonics and treatments. Salesmen traveled from town to town selling actual snake oil claiming it could cure any ailment. There were medical schools, but many were just diploma mills. There were only a small number of good schools in the major cities. Doctors were just one of many competing types of practitioners.

By 1950, America had become increasingly urban and few people had general skills any more. People hired others to do many things that rural people routinely did for themselves.

It had become illegal to practice medicine without a license. This major advance markedly reduced the charlatanism that had victimized so many people in the past. While licensing alone does not guarantee professionalism, physicians had long-standing organizations like the American Medical Association, the American College of Physicians, the American College of Surgeons, and other specialty societies. While part of the function of these groups was to promote and protect the position of physicians, they most importantly set standards, developed codes of ethics, upgraded medical education, and promoted research and patient education.

Critics look at the development of the power of physicians and just see one trade group successfully enhancing its prestige, power, and income by eliminating competition and creating monopolistic control. Sociologist Paul Starr, in his widely acclaimed book *The Social Transformation of American Medicine,* describes this point of view. Milton Friedman, the conservative Chicago economist, is highly critical of licensing, feeling it is monopolistic.

Starr writes that American medicine could have taken a different path. Instead of independent, autonomous practitioners, physicians could have become employees of hospitals and corporations way back in the beginning. Snake oil salesmen, cultists, and anyone else who wanted to could have been allowed to offer medical treatment. Licensing might not have been instituted. Medical schools need not have been restricted to accreditation standards. (Today, medical schools and hospitals must meet strict standards set and enforced by independent agencies.) There used to be diploma mills where any student could get a medical degree with little teaching and no practical experience.

Quite surely, had medicine gone that route, there would be much more competition, much lower cost, and much wider accessibility. The only things lacking would have been skill, quality, knowledge, effectiveness, and value.

We have chosen to promote high standards for many professions, according special privileges and restricting access as the price of quality. We have said that if someone wants to build a bridge, we do not want that bridge to collapse, killing lots of people because the engineer merely paid a fee to obtain his credentials. Few bridges fail today. Engineering standards are very high in this country, in no small measure due to restrictive rules that promote and reward quality.

We want our brightest people to be attracted to professions that are of great value to our country. A smart, highly motivated person is less likely to sacrifice the many years of training needed and to put in the extremely long and hard hours required just to be a low-paid employee of a large corporation. One health economist I spoke with said that when he goes to his own doctor, he *wants* him to be well paid. He wants a happy, well-motivated doctor with a strong interest in succeeding in his care.

For some, the joy of science or the altruistic rewards of medicine might be the only motivation needed, but most people also want the best they can do for themselves. That does not make one any less dedicated, only all the more human.

One can look at the development of American medicine as a sociologist or a theoretical economist and dispassionately postulate ways to save money. We have learned in our country that capitalism, for all its faults, works better than other systems because individuals need the motivation of personal reward to rise to the highest levels of achievement. America has led the world as a virtual cauldron of creativity and productivity in scientific development for just this reason. I hope to successfully show that in the real world, we would sacrifice far more than we would gain if medicine were to be approached in such a manner.

* * *

As the nineteenth century progressed, people turned to doctors more frequently. Physicians could easily be summoned by telephone or telegraph instead of by horseback, which had been the only option in 1850. Radio and later television disseminated information nationally to wide audiences.

Cities began to expand, and people found that urban life was very different from the farm. Adults and children left the house to go to work and to school. Medical care was delivered less and less in the home and increasingly was sought at the doctor's office, clinic, or hospital. House calls were still common, but, as doctors became busier and increasingly dependent on office-based equipment, the home visits became less practical.

While all this increased people's need for doctors, unquestionably the most important reason for the rise of the physician's stature and authority was that, unlike a century before, modern medicine *could* treat and cure disease and relieve suffering! The merging of the ancient arts of healing with the precision and effectiveness of modern science was producing amazing results.

In the Civil War, for example, a blister or a simple wound was frequently a death sentence from infection that could only occasionally be controlled by gruesome amputations. In the Korean War a century later, most soldiers *survived* if they could make it alive to a MASH unit (mobile army surgical hospitals located just behind the battle zone). There were similar, if less dramatic, examples in every aspect of medicine, even as early as 1950.

From the 1920s on, people felt less and less capable or safe in handling their medical problems themselves. The home cures and remedies gave way to doctor appointments. Doctors and hospitals were firmly established as the centers of health care.

Doctors had become honored members of the community, based on an unwritten contract: Doctors gave generously of their time, they treated their patients as the friends and neighbors they usually were, and they employed increasingly effective care. In return, the doctor expected respect, stature in the community, and an affluent lifestyle. Doctors did not expect to get rich, and few did.

By 1960, medicine was a very large part of American life. Hospitals were major forces in society and were huge financial enterprises. Surgery was safer than ever and procedures were becoming very sophisticated. Pharmaceutical companies were developing techniques that would lead to explosive growth in drug treatments. Machines were being invented that could see inside the body in ways X-rays never could. Cardiology was beginning to understand and treat the number-one killer, heart disease. Risk factors for disease were being explored in ways that would lead to effective preventive measures. There were many fine medical schools. As a result the average lifespan increased steadily. People began to feel more secure in their health. It was a golden age in terms of our ability to fight disease and promote health.

In the 1950s, actor Robert Young was America's hero as the television father who knew best (on a show called *Father Knows Best*). It was no accident that by the 1970s, he was the *doctor* who knew best as *Marcus Welby, M.D.*

Television, magazines and newspapers reveled in reporting the real miracles that were coming out of laboratories, research programs, and operating rooms. But as all this was occurring, those seeds of trouble were beginning to grow. In the next chapter we will see how rising costs permitted corporations to grab power and turn proud, autonomous physicians into controlled "providers," not of health care as they claimed, but of corporate profit.

4

Captured by Stealth: How American Business Stole Medicine

The war for freedom will never really be won because the price of freedom is constant vigilance over ourselves and over our government.

—Eleanor Roosevelt

How could anyone steal an industry? Smart businesspeople did just that. They exploited three major developing problems and in the process brought about a radical change in American health care.

The most important problem of which business took advantage was that American society was changing in ways that markedly increased the need for health care and thus its share of resources. The second was the rapidly increasing cost of all the wondrous advances medicine was achieving. The third was that some doctors—by no means the majority—lost touch with the human side of medicine as workloads and incomes rose.

COSTS BEGIN TO ESCALATE

There have been two kinds of cost increases fueling efforts to "reform" health care. The first is the increase in premiums and OOP (out-of-pocket) expenses, which include the deductible, copayment, and whatever is not covered by your policy.

The other cost increase is how much we as a society pay for health care. Health care costs rose from 9 percent of Gross Domestic

Product, (GDP, the cost of all the goods and services sold in that year) in 1980 to 14 percent in 1992. The prediction then was that it would reach 19 percent by year 2000 if trends continued. In 1997, health care costs remained at the 1992 level of 14 percent.

Let us examine premium and OOP expenses.

As surgery and other procedures became more sophisticated, they also became more expensive and more profitable. Hospital costs rose steadily ever higher partly because they were so personnel-intensive, but mostly because of the escalating cost of the new technology and the even bigger expense of caring for the poor and the uninsured who had nowhere else to go. As costs rose, so did the number of people without insurance, which escalated expenditures even further. Medical care delayed is medical cost inflated. Simple, relatively inexpensive treatments begun early can control heart disease, asthma, diabetes, respiratory infections, and many other conditions. But if the diseases are allowed to progress untreated, major complications occur that magnify the cost to sometimes astronomical proportions.

Most uninsured people eventually get care from hospitals (often the emergency ward), which then have to raise their rates, which causes increased insurance premiums, which means more people drop out of insurance, which continues the upward spiral of inflation.

Of course, the tragic health consequences of illness left untreated far outweigh the burden of the costs, but for hospitals, that cost had to be paid for—so they increased costs for the more affluent, insured patients, beyond what was needed to cover their rising expenses. Hospitals then used that excess to pay for the poor and uninsured, education of medical students, and medical research, thus, in effect, imposing a social tax. (Proponents of managed care would later capitalize on this by misleadingly concentrating on a "$5 aspirin tablet" as proof that hospitals were "profiteering.")

Medical costs had already begun to be a significant drain on family budgets by the early part of the century, as people increasingly turned to doctors for help. Various kinds of national health insurance plans had been considered since the 1800s and many European countries established them.

Between 1900 and World War I, unions and socialists made a major effort to pass state and federal compulsory government health insurance. Medical groups, conservatives, insurance companies and large employers all opposed it for their own reasons and little was accomplished.

During Franklin Roosevelt's administration, there were mixed feelings about incorporating health insurance into Social Security.

Some effort was made, but it never went anywhere and the idea was completely abandoned during the preoccupation with World War II.

After the war, President Harry Truman made the most committed effort up to that point, but the same coalition and the rampant anti-communist fervor of the time defeated any effort to pass legislation that seemed even slightly socialist. Public opinion polls showed that the public wanted private insurance, not compulsory public programs.

Doctors' burgeoning prestige, the rapidly increasing demand for their services and the astounding medical advancements they were achieving began to lull some doctors into a sense of infallibility. Doctors could now cure previously fatal infections, operate on living hearts, take over for failing kidneys, vaccinate against more and more diseases, keep diabetics alive, restore vision to many who were previously hopelessly blind, and much more. Some doctors felt the Siren call of wealth and fame. Most doctors continued to practice good, reasonably priced medicine as they always had, but the minority who did not provided ammunition that would later be used to attack the entire profession.

Some doctors succumbed to the temptations of profitable procedures in lucrative specialties. Procedures paid much more and took much less of their time than talking to patients. Surgery; increasingly sophisticated imaging studies; invasive diagnostics like cardiac catheterization, in which tubing could be threaded through arteries in the legs up the heart to do direct tests; endoscopies, in which flexible optical scopes could be inserted to visualize almost the entire gastrointestinal tract; and other procedures gradually became a major factor in physician billing, escalating costs ever higher. For example, in the same amount of time an internist might spend seeing a patient for hypertension, a gastroenterologist might do a colonoscopy. The internist might charge, say, $60 for the visit while the colonoscopy would be billed for $600, ten times the amount of money for a procedure that took the same amount of face-to-face (so to speak) patient contact. Despite overhead costs for the procedure, the profit margin was very high. We will discuss later how to value medical services, but for now it is reasonable to say that to some degree the office visit was undervalued and the procedure overvalued.

PRIVATE HEALTH INSURANCE

Patients at first did not perceive the increased costs directly because most were absorbed by health insurance. They did begin to feel it in their premiums.

Insurance companies had avoided offering health insurance for a very long time, having correctly perceived the unpredictability of risk in health care. They feared becoming caught in a quicksand of escalating costs. They were correct, but eventually found a way around it.

The Great Depression that began in 1929 had hit doctors and hospitals as hard as it hit the jobless. Patients could not pay their bills. My father entered private practice in the depth of the Depression. He was lucky to get one dollar for an office visit and two dollars for a house call. Often he was paid in eggs or a piece of chicken or he saw the patient for free.

A private group of community and medical leaders known as the Committee on the Costs of Medical Care met in 1929. Their work and the work of others led to the development of Blue Cross to pay for hospital bills and later Blue Shield for doctor bills. This was important not just for the coverage these insurance plans provided, but because the system that developed would change medical care dramatically and set in place practices that persist to this day.

The committee's original fee schedules (what was to be paid for by the insurance and at what rate per procedure) set a pattern whose flaws were not recognized until much later, when it was too late. Procedures were reimbursed at much higher rates than cognitive care (the general term for patient care that does not involve a procedure, such as talking to a patient, thinking about the problem, and prescribing medication). Billing was based on units, such as visits, tests, and procedures, unlike the legal profession, which bills for the time spent at an hourly rate with no limits. The effect of unit pricing and favoring procedures was to reward doing something to a patient and to make spending time and thought on a patient economically less desirable. This time bomb would later wreak great havoc as procedures became much more profitable than cognitive care.

TWO APPROACHES TO INSURANCE DEVELOPMENT

There are two basic ways to insure health care: *indemnity* and *direct service*.

Originally, Blue Cross and Blue Shield were indemnity plans, which means that they contracted with the patient (or more usually the patient's employer) to reimburse a predetermined percentage of all medical bills for services covered under the plan. In indemnity plans, the insurer has no relationship with the doctor or hospital. The patient chooses his or her care and is billed directly. The patient is responsible for paying the bill and then obtaining reimbursement from the insurer.

Direct service is just the opposite. The insurance company contracts with the physicians and the hospitals of *its* choice to provide care to the patient, who pays a premium to the insurance company for using their services. All managed care plans are of this latter type, which will be discussed shortly.

Blue Cross and Blue Shield began selling indemnity insurance to employers for their employees. The companies either paid the premium in full as an employee benefit or charged for it by a payroll deduction. This was great for employees lucky enough to work for such companies. They got free insurance or, most often, much cheaper group rates. The employers saw it as a benefit to either discourage unionization, or, if too late, to assuage other union concerns. The unions recognized it as an important benefit, though at first they feared it might diminish their influence since many unions were already involved in trying to provide for their members. Hospitals and doctors saw it as a way to broaden accessibility to health care to those in need, to increase their patient base, and to remove pressures on their own pricing.

Private insurance companies recognized the employer-based system as the solution to their concerns. They would not need an army of agents selling door to door; they would just have to sell a single policy to an employer. By spreading risk over a large pool of people they could better predict risk and keep premiums reasonable.

What could go wrong with such a great system that made everybody happy? What went wrong is that no one was watching the costs.

Insurance companies were just cashiers, taking the money in and handing it out, after deducting their administrative costs and profit. As costs went up, they were simply passed along to the employers/employees in the form of higher premiums.

Patients did not feel the the full brunt of bills because they only paid a small percentage of them. Every patient wanted the best care that someone else's money could buy.

Doctors could remain concerned with giving the best care. It was great that they could give the patient everything the patient needed without having to worry about what it cost and they could raise their fees as they wished. Just as happily, the more physicians did for the benefit of the patient the more they also did for their own incomes. In the early years the employer companies that could afford to offer such insurance plans were large enough that the premiums were at first not high enough to concern them. Besides, at the time, they were preoccupied with their union relationships.

Everybody was happy until the costs began to rise high enough that premiums became painful. Patients began to feel it in two ways. First, their payroll deductions became very noticeable. Then their copayments began to increase noticeably. Twenty percent of a $100 bill is a lot less painful than 20 percent of a $1,000 bill.

Insurance deductibles began to rise as insurers decided to stop paying 80 percent of the bill. Instead, they paid 80 percent of the "allowed" amount for that service. The allowed amount was based on what they described as the "usual and customary charges based on a broad sample of prevailing fees," or some variant thereof. They set their own limits on what they would pay for each procedure as they saw fit and used the euphemism of "usual and customary" to deflect criticism to the doctors. If a doctor charged more than the insurance carrier allowed, it looked like he was charging more than anyone else was. The patients did not know how artificial the insurance company limits were.

Thus, the doctor might bill $100. The insurance company would allow $80 and then pay 80 percent of that, which would be $64. The patient's out-of-pocket cost (what the patient actually had to pay in cash) would thus be the remaining $36, which amounted to a copayment of 36 percent instead of the promised 20 percent. In this way, the out-of-pocket costs for patients and the insurance costs for the employer began to rise rapidly and often considerably faster than overall inflation. The insurance companies were not affected because they simply passed the costs on to their customers.

Doctors and hospitals at first felt no pain because the services they provided were so essential and desirable that they were utilized despite the cost. Also there was little incentive for doctors and hospitals to control costs or eliminate waste. Patients were demanding more and more care. The media's fascination with everything medical and all the newest wonders pushed demand higher and higher. The more glorious the success stories, the more people expected miraculous results. Patients were armed with increasingly informed requests for the newest and the best treatments and procedures. The stage was set and something had to give. People and companies were complaining bitterly and doctors were paying no heed.

Had costs increased gradually, people would have adjusted. What sparked the resentment was the rapidity of the change that did not allow people in effect to reset their financial thermostat. We have weathered increases in costs for many things in daily life without complaint, but rapid change always causes strain.

Before we discuss what occurred next, it is important to understand two other important developments: the beginnings of direct service insurance and Medicare.

MEDICARE BECOMES LAW

In 1963, an assassin's bullet brought to the presidency a man such as the office had rarely seen before. Lyndon Johnson was a natural force of tornado proportions. Recently released tapes and a biography by Doris Kearns Goodwin[1] reveal a man of such powerful personality and conviction that few could resist him. He was also something no other president in this century was—a master of the Congress.

In 1965, Johnson and the Democratic majority he brought with him in his landslide victory accomplished what had never been done before—they passed two national health insurance programs, Medicare and Medicaid. As lifespan lengthened, there were increasing numbers of people over sixty-five and they used hospitals and doctors at a much higher rate than younger people did. There was strong political support for this age group. People over age sixty-five hold a major portion of the nation's wealth. Although some of that is in non-liquid assets, such as homes, many have adequate funds or are affluent. However, more than half of this age group have only Social Security or small pensions for support or limited savings that will not be replenished in retirement. Members of this latter group are in great difficulty because their monthly income lags far behind inflation's impact over the years. Medical expenses consume a major portion of their budgets.

The original concept behind Medicare and Medicaid was to provide assistance only for those in need, but such a limited approach would not fly politically. There were objections to means testing (using income levels to determine eligibility) as demeaning and there was concern that it would lead to extending expensive coverage to all needy people. Some wanted coverage for hospital bills, others for doctor bills. The final result was a political compromise. *Medicare* would be a program available to *all* people over sixty-five, the Social Security retirement age. It was divided into a mandatory Part A for hospital bills and a voluntary Part B for doctor bills. To avoid the appearance of direct government bureaucracy, "carriers" were authorized as intermediaries—Blue Cross and Blue Shield in most cases.

Medicaid was enacted at the same time to provide for the poor under the age of sixty-five. Medicare was relatively generous direct payment with very loose controls. Medicaid was administered through limited grants to the states and entailed very tight controls.

Medicare differed from traditional insurance. It did not indemnify in the usual way nor did it employ physicians or hospitals. It simply used the power of the federal government to impose price controls on every physician and hospital in the country. It set fees far below the prevailing rates and established rules that at first were limited, but later grew to fill over *thirty thousand pages* and continues to expand.

Medicare eventually changed the landscape as dramatically as an earthquake. Doctors were very resistant at first, until they discovered the stream of newly empowered Medicare patients knocking on their doors. The fees were lower but the volume was higher. It was also very satisfying to finally be able to help people in great need who previously had avoided medical care because of the costs.

There were more time bombs in the wings, waiting to explode, however. Medicine had begun as a doctor taking care of a patient and being paid in return. When third parties—the insurance companies and the government—entered the transaction, the whole doctor-patient relationship began to change. Gradually, payments began to come from the insurer, not the patient. That alone is a big difference, even if the third party is the insurance company as a disinterested "cashier" or if it is the government. Interest shifted to the needs of the payer rather than those of the patient seeking care.

Economic transactions work best when the party most interested in the result is also the party that pays the bill. If you want to buy a refrigerator, you will look hard for the best one at a price you can afford. If someone else is paying the bill for you, but you get to choose which one, you will choose the most expensive brand possible.

Medicare and Medicaid bureaucrats began to insert themselves into the doctor-patient relationship and impose mandatory rules. Under private insurance, doctors could choose whether to participate. A doctor seeing a patient under Medicare or Medicaid had no choice but to abide by the rules and fee structure or forego those patients. Since virtually *all* patients over sixty-five came under Medicare, it was either submit to the government or give up a major portion of the practice. Pediatricians were the only doctors initially unaffected.

The change in focus from doctor control to third party control began to subtly affect patients' perceptions of the profession. The low Medicare fees fueled non-Medicare patients' distrust of doctors.

Patients assumed that the government fees must be all the doctor deserved and therefore anything higher was an overcharge. Patients began to sense the doctor's diminished authority. Gradually, the Medicare model influenced all insurance coverage.

THE BEGINNINGS OF MANAGED CARE

Prepaid medical care for a group began as far back as the 1800s when some slaveholders realized that healthy slaves were better workers. They arranged with local doctors to form a medical group that gave rudimentary care to the slaves, enough to keep them working. Fortunately, modern corporations have not gone quite that far.[2] Later, some ethnic groups like orthodox Jews created medical groups that would respect the strict requirements of their religion.

These were all minor developments until the 1940s, when some major plans began. Two of the largest were the Kaiser-Permanente plan in the West and the HIP (Health Insurance Plan) in New York. Both continue to this day. When they began they were nonprofit, idealistic attempts to bring affordable quality health care and preventive advice to people who might not have access to such care. They were seen as an ideal way to contain costs within reasonable bounds while maintaining quality of care.

Kaiser and HIP are primarily staff model health maintenance organizations (HMOs). Patients are seen at the HMO facility by doctors who work there on salary. The other model consists of patients who are seen by their doctor in his own office, but the bills are paid by the insurer under contracts between the doctor and the insurer.

Kaiser and HIP are nonprofit. That means that they operate on funds that are used for operating their business; they do not pay dividends to stockholders or make distributions to investors. They devote a higher percentage of their premiums to patient care than do for-profits. They can be very profitable to the executives, who are often paid high salaries. They apply the same methods as for-profit companies, but with somewhat different allocations.

I have observed some HMO clinics, though by no means can I offer a comprehensive survey. The buildings ranged from nice to magnificent and the full-time doctors were paid good to very high salaries, with great benefits. All that was usually missing was the patient care.

In facilities I observed, doctors saw as many as ten patients per hour, despite the fact that most of the patients were in great need of comprehensive care. Many of the patients were lower income; long underserved elsewhere; and sadly, treated no better at these clinics. When I made recommendations, such as spending more time with patients, I was told my suggestions were "luxuries we cannot afford."

Health maintenance organizations are an assembly-line type of care in which the process of handling large numbers seems overwhelming and the results run contrary to the quality patient care HMOs allegedly seek. Clinics by their nature serve a large volume of patients. It takes great vigilance to avoid losing sight of priorities. Some succeed, but many do not.

I currently see patients a few days a week in a well-funded primary care clinic for low-income patients in need. This clinic allows time for patient care and the goal is quality, not volume. Thus, high-quality care is provided. However, when my clinic patients need tests or consultations outside of the clinic, their only choice is a hospital clinic or emergency room. The difference in treatment is shockingly apparent, because such facilities are usually so overloaded that there is little time or inclination to provide personal care. It is frustrating to see how frequently those in greatest need are not given quality care.

HIP and Kaiser were the forerunners of managed care, but they and other HMOs have changed dramatically, as we will see when we discuss today's managed care.

DOCTORS ARE AFFECTED

Most doctors responded to the shifts in insurance coverage with great frustration and unhappiness. The initial euphoria with the early windfall Medicare provided was eventually dissipated by the hidden price. These hidden costs—the loss of autonomy, the damage to relationships with patients, and much more—will be covered in depth in chapters 5 and 6.

Despite these problems, most physicians did not reduce the care of their patients. Most simply continued to practice medicine the same as they always had and spent time with patients even if they were not compensated for the extra effort.

Changes continued at faster and faster rates:

- Technology was developing new medical procedures at an astonishing pace. For example, the only treatment for coronary artery disease, where blood flow to the heart is impaired, used to be a drug called nitroglycerin. Now there are dozens of medical treatments and many kinds of procedures to open the blockage or bypass it.

- Society was telling medicine that it only cared about what could be concretely counted. Insurance companies and the government began to monitor doctors increasingly intrusively and to do so, came to value only what could be recorded and tabulated.
- Spurred by media fascination with perceived miracles and new technology, patients expected more and more and only the newest and the best would do.
- The insurance shifts were inducing an adversarial tone into patient care because doctors increasingly were caught between patient demands and insurance company and government limitations.
- Pressures on fees intensified as insurers and the government sought to contain costs by reducing payments to doctors.

As the field of medicine became bigger and more complex, it became much harder to keep track of medical procedures. For example, outmoded procedures such as preventive routine tonsillectomies and various treatments that proved useless or harmful persisted beyond any reasonable time needed to recognize their faults.

In a free market, prices are set by supply and demand. In a regulated market or where the supplier makes the rules, normal market forces no longer apply. As government and insurance companies set fees and regulations, they controlled the market for medical care, but there were unexpected results. For example, tempted by the high incomes and glory, the number of surgeons trained continued to increase, although there was no increased need for surgery. Some surgeons were popular and overworked but the others did fewer and fewer procedures. So they charged *more* to make up for the reduced volume.

Physicians still enjoyed a very high prestige and approval rating into the 1980s, but the increasing power of the government and insurance companies would light a fuse on an economic bomb that would soon explode.

THE MOST IMPORTANT REASON COSTS WENT UP

The discovery of how much health care was costing became almost a mantra—"Health care costs are eating up 14 percent of GDP and will soon consume 100 percent of everything we own or will ever have."

Every news outlet repeated the same figures and outcry. The public was led to believe that doctors were completely responsible for the high prices and rapidly rising cost of health care. Making the doctors the culprits paved the way for the takeover by insurers that was to come.

In truth, doctors account for only a modest portion of health costs. As the putative captains of the medical ship, however, they are supposed to be accountable for all that occurs. In reality, doctors were gradually being demoted to little more than deck hands, but the public was led to believe that the high prices and low-quality care were their fault.

It is true that doctors were slow to recognize the impact of increased costs, and their role in those costs. It is equally true that they did not themselves make a major effort to eliminate waste and to put reasonable limits on use of procedures. It is also true that some doctors overcharged and that some fees were too high. These were major failures on the part of the medical profession.

Having said all this, the reality is that waste, inefficiency, and excessive fees were but a drop in the bucket compared to the *real* cause of the "crisis" in medical costs, which had become the rallying cry of the 1980s.

In the final chapter, we will discuss at length how much of our resources *should* be devoted to health. For now let us examine some of the factors that make medical costs so high:

- In the thirty years since I graduated from the Columbia University College of Physicians and Surgeons, the United States population has grown by *65 million* people! This is like annexing the population of France and Finland to our own. It costs a lot to provide health care for another two nations!
- The population has aged tremendously. There are already nearly four million people aged eighty-five or older and their numbers will skyrocket in coming years. While older people are healthier than before, they still need health resources many times more (and more often) than younger people.
- We are suffering new waves of infectious disease, such as AIDS and chronic hepatitis, which are very expensive diseases to treat.
- As people live longer, chronic diseases like heart disease and cancer increase in frequency. New technologies have ballooned the cost of treating these diseases.
- Wholly new technologies like transplantation, coronary bypass and angioplasty, survival care of babies as premature as only 24

weeks, advanced intensive care techniques, dialysis, and medicinal preventive care (such as antihypertension and cholesterol lowering drugs) added enormous cost.

- Massive waves of illegal immigrants bring new, highly needy consumers of health care who require public support—over 2 million in California alone—costing billions.[3]
- New technologies in every area are turning simple treatments into highly expensive enterprises. For example, it used to cost $150 to X-ray a head injury. A head X-ray is now obsolete and virtually constitutes malpractice because a $1,000 magnetic residence imaging scan of the brain is so much better. MRI is a space-age technology that uses computers, radio waves, and giant magnets to give incredibly detailed pictures of the body's interior. An X-ray cannot see blood on the brain; an MRI can detect even tiny amounts of bleeding.
- The increasing numbers of uninsured people magnify costs because, as noted previously, they still get care, but delayed, which is much more costly.
- The poor and uninsured use emergency rooms for routine care, which is inefficient and very expensive.
- Poverty is increasing as the gap between rich and poor steadily widens. Poverty breeds medical expense because poor nutrition, substandard living conditions, and lack of medical and preventive care markedly increase the likelihood of serious illness.
- Social inequity persists as people of color continue to receive inferior care due to social factors such as lower income and discrimination, which reduce access to health care and education. Inferior care is very expensive because the resulting poor outcomes are much more expensive to treat than they would have been to prevent.

There is another important factor. Former U.S. Surgeon General C. Everett Koop was asked who was more greedy, doctors or hospitals? (The question itself was terrible and illustrated the depths to which the medical image has fallen.) Dr. Koop said that the answer was neither—the greediest were the *patients*. He meant that we all want the very best health care for ourselves that other people's money can buy, as long as *we* do not have to pay for it.

PRESIDENT CLINTON TRIES

In January 1993, Bill Clinton took office as president. The crown jewel of his administration was to be a national health care plan that would solve the endemic problems and give excellent care to every citizen. By fall of 1993, the plan was presented to the public, but it found no political following and soon died.

What went wrong?

The president appointed his wife, Hillary, to head the health care effort. She is a very bright and organized lawyer but she had not had experience in health care. Mrs. Clinton hired Ira Magaziner, an analyst, to run the program. Magaziner was well known for a number of studies. Articles in popular publications criticized his previous efforts in which he had brought together large numbers of planners and developed enormously complex plans that then fizzled.

Whether the articles about his previous efforts were correct or not, that is exactly what happened in the case of national health care. The White House recruited over five hundred alleged experts from think tanks, universities, politics, large medical institutions, and so on. The participants' names were kept secret at the time, as were their deliberations, in order, it was said, to avoid lobbying and other interference in their work.

No one bothered to include real doctors in practice, real people who were patients, real mothers whose only constituency was their own family. They did read sad letters from people who had problems under the current system, however. There were few, if any, physicians, and those represented large organizations. I do not believe physicians who are not in full private practice can fully represent the views of those doctors who are.

This special group did not work with the existing system to ensure that there would be a smooth transition and that those who would lose under the new system, such as doctors and the indemnity insurance industry, would be compensated in some way so as to help win their cooperation.

In the end, *Health Security, the President's Report to the American People* was published in October 1993.[4] The report claimed that the excess cost of health care (that which exceeded what the commission claimed the cost would have been if reform had been instituted in 1975) reduced the average wage earner's annual income by $1,000, and another $600 by the year 2000. "Health Security" (trying to capture the aura of everybody's favorite, Social Security) became the new euphemism.

The commission claimed, with little documentation, that quality of care was low and that we paid much more for much less care than other countries do. The report described the problems of the uninsured, the limitations of managed care, the high administrative costs and much more. Some of their observations were correct and others were off base.

The proposed solution was to impose a national health plan guaranteeing every American basic health coverage from a variety of sources. Administrative functions would be simplified and centralized, there would be no exclusions for pre-existing conditions, and so on. Central agencies would set national standards and guidelines, as well as fees and other financial aspects.

Though I looked carefully throughout the report, listened to the enormous publicity campaign, and read the public relations releases and the endless media reporting, I never found one mention of the central assumption of the plan: doctors' fees and procedures would be fixed and dictated by the government. In effect, the entire physician workforce was being secretly conscripted to be employees of the government, whether they wanted to or not. Long after the plan died, supporters claimed that doctors would have been free to see patients privately, but even if this were technically correct, the plan would have so monopolized health care that in practice doctors would have been employees.

This concept was not very popular with doctors, but by this time it seemed as if they were minor figures in health care. They had not been included in the planning and they were the invisible people in the health care reform debate.

Doctors are not well organized and are not used to waging public relations campaigns. They work sixty- to seventy-hour weeks doing unimportant things like treating diseases and saving lives. The AMA, which now represents far fewer doctors than in the past, was once a powerful lobby, but while it still spends heavily, it is being outgunned more and more.

The insurance industry, however, are masters at public relations and are known for mounting highly successful advertising blitzes to change the public and Congress's views.

The Health Insurance Association of America (HIAA), the powerful trade group well-funded by the managed care insurers, spent over $14 million on an ad campaign featuring a husband and wife, Harry and

Louise, who expressed middle-class dismay over the provisions of the proposal. The campaign received enormous attention and was a major factor in shifting public opinion against health security legislation.

The public seemed to understand that this plan would have brought the government into their homes and doctor visits, and they felt uncomfortable with it. Little did they know that the sponsors of the ads were wolves in sheep's clothing and that American families would be the next meal.

Politically, Congress worried about the enormous cost of the plan and members were skeptical of the estimates of the savings promised to offset the budget-busting cost of putting the health care system into place and maintaining it. Senator Arlen Spector (R-Penn.) stunned his fellow legislators when he diagrammed the Rube Goldberg-esque bureaucracy needed to implement the president's plan.

Betsey McCaughey Ross (then an analyst with the free-market Manhattan Institute think tank who later became Lieutenent Governor of New York) wrote a cover story in the then Clinton-friendly *New Republic,* claiming that she had read the entire Clinton plan. She concluded in annotated and excruciating detail that it repeatedly contradicted itself. She later went on to win a national magazine award for her analysis.

The plan died quickly and no further government ideas were offered to replace it until 1997, when the administration began to propose piecemeal programs for select groups. What they couldn't achieve as a whole, Clinton aides felt, they could possibly secure as separate, smaller, more manageable pieces of legislation.

FILLING A VACUUM

The Clinton plan had painted a dismal picture of an American medical system that it hoped to reform. While all this legislative haggling was taking place, doctors went right on treating their patients as usual, but they did not fully realize how much their image had deteriorated in the public's mind.

Costs continued to increase at rates well in excess of inflation. Insurance premiums increased steadily. It was my impression at the time that the premiums were increasing much faster than costs. The general assumption was that it was the fault of those greedy doctors.

I think doctors were unfairly accused. Physician fees are only 20

TABLE 4.1

UNITED STATES HEALTH COSTS 1995 BY CATEGORY

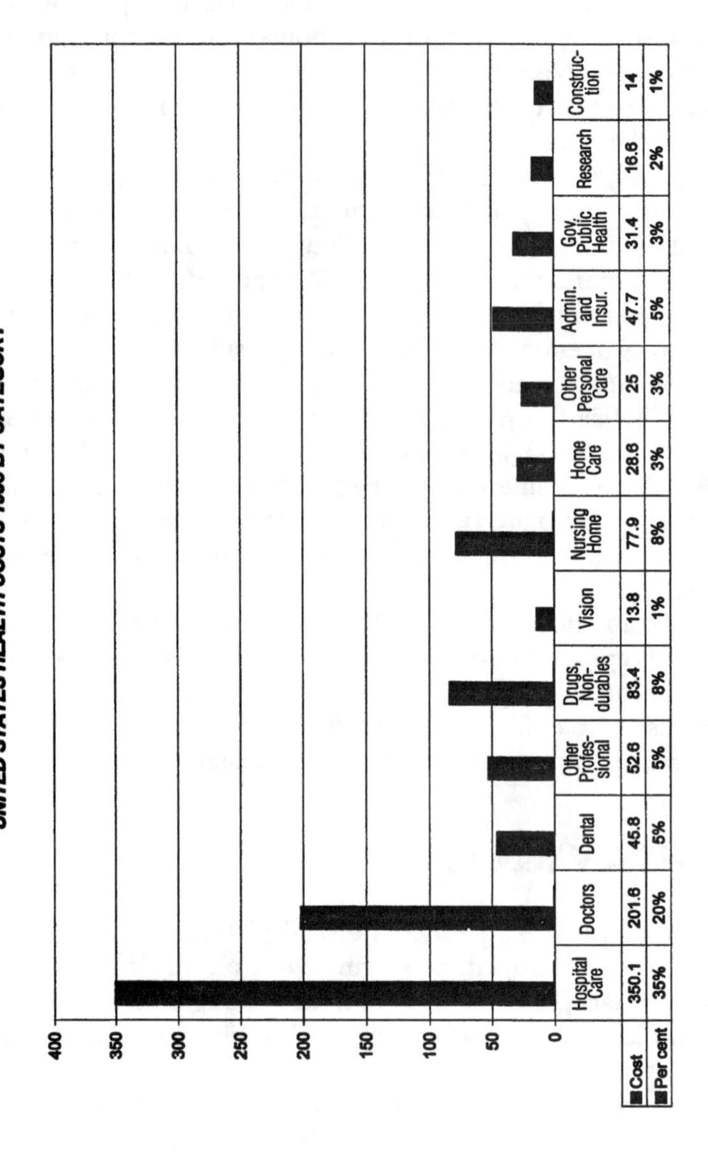

	Hospital Care	Doctors	Dental	Other Profes-sional	Drugs, Non-durables	Vision	Nursing Home	Home Care	Other Personal Care	Admin. and Insur.	Gov. Public Health	Research	Construc-tion
Cost	350.1	201.6	45.8	52.6	83.4	13.8	77.9	28.6	25	47.7	31.4	16.6	14
Per cent	35%	20%	5%	5%	8%	1%	8%	3%	3%	5%	3%	2%	1%

Adapted from John W. Wright (ed.), *The New York Times 1998 Almanac* (New York: Penguin Group, 1997), p. 382.

percent of health costs (see table 4.1)* and doctors influence a much smaller portion of costs than in the past. There were many factors pushing up costs, including administrative costs due to the insurance companies and the government, insurance companies' profits, the increasing expense for medications and for providing long-term care, and the hidden but huge amount of money being channeled into the coffers of those who provide alternative medicine.

Another important factor was that managed care plans were draining off inexpensive, young, healthy subscribers, forcing indemnity insurers to raise the premiums for their remaining policy holders, who tended to incur more health care expense.

The media that had delighted in singing the praises of medical miracles and caring doctors now began to write about costs, greed, uncaring doctors, and health care fraud. There was no discussion about how much we should pay for health care or how we should allocate our resources (a subject we will cover in the last chapter). If prices were going up, no one seemed to notice that there were good reasons, they just assumed that the costs, whatever they were, must be too high! Costs were high, but not as high as the passions about them. Pressure for limiting fees and costs under the banner of health care "reform" became even more intense.

The main force for change was, and still is, unrecognized. The real engine for change was behind the scenes. Behind it lay the fact that Wall Street financing and dynamics had changed radically in the 1980s. The price of a company's stock became more important than its performance. Prior to the 1980s there was a relatively direct relationship between company performance and the price of its stock for most companies. Bonds were solid, secure investments, inflation was in single digits, and the main market was the New York Stock Exchange. Then inflation during the Carter administration soared into the high teens and remained high into the early 1980s.

Wall Street began a radical transformation with mergers and acquisitions fueled by a new device called junk bonds. Financial transactions fragmented to many different kinds of markets. Computers permitted stock purchasing based on market performance more than on company performance. All of this brought huge fortunes to big players that then further fueled the acceleration of financial power. Executive salaries also rose to much higher levels than ever before.

---

*Table 4.1 does not reflect total administrative costs under the category "Administration and Insurance." Administrative costs are a large portion of every category.

At the same time, America was beginning to transform from a manufacturing and industrial economy to a service and information economy. Corporations, utilizing computer technology, grew ever larger and more powerful. The mergers and acquisitions began to concentrate power in fewer and fewer hands.

This had several effects on health care. First of all, executives at all companies felt enormous pressure from Wall Street to show steady increase in earning and profit. Also, the same pressures for size and consolidation of power affected insurance companies and large health care entities as well.

Another important factor was that executives, criticized for high salaries, wanted to find less obvious compensation. Thus was born the era of stock options. Offering executives the opportunity to purchase stock at a fixed price even when the value of the stock is much higher can be a lucrative component of any compensation package. These incentives are not new and have been a great way for start-up companies to attract talented people. If their efforts pay off and the company stock goes way up, they stand to benefit enormously. It's an incentive to be creative and to succeed. However, stock options now became very popular among executives as a way to soften the appearance of large compensation packages. For example, Norman Payson, when he was the head of an HMO called Healthsource, could say he made a salary of only $387,604 plus a few stock options, but those options were worth $15.1 million![5]

Thus began the enormous pressure on executives to maximize the appearance of the bottom line and to produce apparent steady growth that would fuel stock price increases and incidentally make executive stock options more lucrative. This was great for stockholders and is probably one reason for the remarkable bull market Wall Street has experienced. (Whether it was good for everyone else, such as the victims of downsizing and the neighborhood stores forced to close by the seemingly endless march of large chains, is an argument for another time and another volume.)

How do shifts in financial practices relate to health care reform? A major drain on the bottom line is the cost of providing health insurance for employees. Stories began to appear in the media that workers' health insurance added $400 to $700 to the cost of every car made in the United States. That was supposed to be much more than in Japan, and the extra cost was said to be making it hard for us to compete with the Japanese cars that were undermining sales of domestic cars. The problems of American automakers had a lot more to do with the fact that, at that time, Japanese cars were much *better* than theirs were, but the health insurance cost factor sounded impressive. Since then, the Japanese have begun to manufacture many more cars in the United States, and America has learned from them how to make quality cars. We are now very competitive even though recently General Motors claimed that the added cost of providing health coverage to its workers is now $1,200 per car!

The old saying is that there are lies, damned lies, and statistics. To that, we might add corporate accounting tricks. For one thing, the money GM pays for employee health insurance is deductible. For another, if GM did not provide such coverage, it would still be paying that money in the form of higher salaries (so the cars would not cost less). If their employees did not have health insurance, GM would suffer productivity losses from an unhealthy workforce. The company simply made medical costs the scapegoat for its own failure to produce competitve cars.

Since large corporations found themselves having to provide health insurance as a part of their employee salary and benefits package, they wanted to find ways to do so at much less cost. So they began exerting enormous pressure and sought out managed care solutions to their health insurance costs.[6] General Motors and the rest of corporate America would have liked nothing better than to shift the increasing burden of health costs. They could not shift costs to the government, however, because it would just increase taxes to pay the extra cost. And the insurance companies would just fight back.

Paul Ellwood, a pediatric neurologist, had long theorized that the solution to the alleged quality problems in health care could be solved by managing health care. He is given the credit for coining the term "Health Maintenance Organization." He felt that doctors needed help in determining which treatments and tests were effective and which were not. He wanted to find ways to increase preventive care and to reduce wasteful and counterproductive practices. He believed that competition and empowered health care insurers could accomplish this by managed care. Ellwood himself has since said in effect that his plans were subverted.[7]

However, early on he succeeded, with others, in convincing the Nixon administration that HMOs were the answer. This resulted in the HMO Act of 1973, which legitimized HMOs, created seed grants, and empowered and promoted HMOs in various ways. It accomplished its goal and HMOs began to grow.

Initially, HMOs began as nonprofit institutions. Then they started to seek more capital so they could expand and spread their message.

The best place to raise capital is Wall Street, but to do so the HMOs would have to forego their nonprofit status. Gradually, the nonprofits began to convert to for-profit corporations (often having to compensate the community by setting aside money for health prevention foundations). They were very successful and raised large sums when they sold stock on the public exchanges.

The early HMOs had been run more as noble missions with frugal budgets and modest salaries. Another incentive to convert was that going public meant huge windfalls to the executives who had previously worked for modest compensation.[8]

While becoming a publicly traded company can provide a huge capital infusion, going public also means that a company has to please investors or the stock price falls. To please investors, the company has to show increasing profits and a promising business strategy. Thus began a major change in health care delivery. The only way to increase profits is to decrease costs, and the savings have to come from the customers, which are you and your family. *You* became the vehicle for stock market success.

The HMOs would have to fool you and your employers, because you would be very unhappy to learn that you were just a pawn in a financial game. Thus began all the theories and propaganda about how reducing your health benefits is actually good for you.

HMOs quickly achieved high-level penetration in a few areas, including Minnesota and parts of California, but the growth was slow. Few people expected places like New York to be affected.

In the meantime, businesspeople were looking around and saw that there was tremendous profit potential in managed care. Health care had become very big business and they wanted a share of it. The HMOs and the hospitals ripe for corporate takeovers were the perfect answer. As managed care companies became successful, they began to acquire and merge with other companies. This significantly increased the power of the companies to deal with businesses and to force their way on the health care industry. By reducing premium levels they could attact more and more client companies whose workforce would be young enough not to pose a significant threat to the HMO's expenses through care delivery.

By 1994 there was a void left by the failure of the Clinton health care reform plan. The managed care companies were ready. The major corporate employers were demanding a solution to rising health insurance premiums.

Onto the stage stepped budding managed care companies, corporations looking for a way to reduce their payroll costs and businessmen seeking gold by tapping into the huge health care market. Thus was born *managed cost.*

What Paul Ellwood and others had intially envisioned as a way to improve the quality and cost effectiveness of health care became instead a means of reducing costs for corporations through lower employee premiums and producing income for managed care executives.

Where would the savings and profits come from? From the two weakest players in the game: patients and doctors. Corporations could now improve their bottom line by shifting more and more of the cost of health care from their budgets to the pocketbooks of their employees. It worked wonderfully:

- In the beginning, coporations had paid their employees' health insurance premiums or at least subsidized them. As premiums increased, workers had to pay more of the cost themselves. Under managed care, those premium costs for employees of small businesses went up many multiples over the past decade and as much as 21 percent just in the last year, while their employers' costs stayed even or perhaps dropped a little lower.[9] The companies passed the increases on to the employees, keeping their own costs down.
- Taxpayers are picking up an increasing percentage of the costs as managed care shifts sicker people into public programs.[10] This occurs because those needing the most care lose their insurace and end up either on Medicaid or in hospital clinics and emergency rooms.
- People are paying much higher out-of-pocket costs as managed care increasingly restricts what it will cover.[11]

Managed care claims to be reducing costs, but what it actually does is take money from doctors by forcing them into low-paying contracts and from patients by reducing benefits and increasing out-of-pocket costs. The money that was supposed to be used to help people now goes for executives' salaries, high administrative costs, and very healthy profits. As managed care spread, doctors could either join or lose many of their patients.

Where the original nonprofit HMOs took only 5 to 10 percent of premiums for administration and income, for-profit HMOs take as high as *over 30* percent for administration, salaries, and profits. Managed care had won over government and business, now it had to lull the public into thinking this was good for them.

Wonderful commercials appeared about the golden old days of ice cream and kites, doctors in buggies making house calls, beautiful children looking trustingly at a white-coated doctor, nostalgic music. The commercials cloaked managed care with images stolen from the glory of the very system that their business practices were in effect busily destroying.

The media loved the companies. Premium increases were slowing and they had a great fall guy in the rich, greedy doctor image they had created. Wall Street was happy and many managed care executives got incredibly rich. In fact, everyone was happy, except doctors and sick people. Before anyone noticed, the momentum was unstoppable.

Insurance succeeds by spreading the risk (the potential for financial loss caused by sickness, flood, fire, or whatever else is being insured against) over a large pool, limiting the cost for each participant. The larger the pool, the less the cost for each individual. As employers jumped at the chance to reduce their premiums by switching to cheaper managed care contracts, more people came under managed care and fewer were in the traditional insurance pools.

That drove up the price of traditional insurance, which drove more people into managed care. The cycle continued until traditional insurance became all but extinct in many parts of the country. Managed care now has over 85 percent of employment-based insurance and a rising percentage of everything else. Because of this, the cost of traditional insurance has *doubled!*

Many doctors joined HMOs early to avoid being left out of what they saw as an inevitable transformation. Some recognized that they could profit more under managed care than previously if they adapted to the system. Some became executives of managed care companies and made tens of millions of dollars per year, as did business people in many companies. The *Wall Street Journal* headlined the story, "Penny-Pinching H.M.O.'s Showed Their Generosity in Executive Paychecks," as shown in table 4.2.

As the companies were denying care to their customers, sometimes causing unnecessary suffering, injury, and even death, the executives were pocketing millions of dollars and building palatial homes and offices.[12] Many of the companies made such huge profits that they had as much as $1 billion in cash they did not know how to spend. This was occuring at a time that they were refusing to pay their policyholders many important benefits that had previously been well established under traditional insurance.[13] The denial of benefits is discussed in the chapters on problems of managed care and in many of the references, such as George Anders's book, *Health against Wealth.*

TABLE 4.2

Executive	Company	1994 Compensation
Norman C. Payson, M.D.	Healthsource	$15,500,000
Daniel D. Crowley	Foundation Health	$13,700,000
Roger F. Greaves	Health Systems International	$ 8,900,000
Malik M. Hasan, M.D.	Health Systems International	$ 8,800,000
William W. McGuire, M.D.	United Healthcare	$ 6,800,000
Leonard Abramson	U.S. Healthcare	$ 3,900,000
George T. Jochum	Mid Atlantic Medical Services	$ 3,700,000
Stephen F. Wiggins	Oxford Health Plans	$ 2,800,000

Adapted from Milt Freudenheim, "Penny-Pinching H.M.O.'s Showed Their Generosity in Executive Paychecks," *Wall Street Journal* (April 11, 1995), D4.

The insurance industry uses a term called the medical-loss ratio, as Anders describes in his book. The medical-loss ratio is the percentage of premiums collected that are paid out to subscribers as benefits, expressed as a percentage. For example, if a company takes in $1 billion in premiums and pays out $900 million to reimburse health care expenses of its customers, that would be a medical-loss ratio of 90 percent. That means the company would spend 90 percent on benefits and keep 10 percent ($100 million) for itself.

Traditional non-profit HMOs in the past had ratios of 95 percent, meaning that they spent 95 percent of the monies they collected to pay for subscribers' health bills. In contrast, the medical-loss ratios at HMOs that are run for profit have been as low as 68 percent![14] Such a company would spend only 68 percent of the money it took in for subscribers' medical bills and it would keep the other 32 percent for itself to pay for those huge executive salaries, fancy buildings, stockholder dividends, and the army of overseers who control the doctors in the network.

Anders notes that the companies took what had been an accounting term and turned it into a goal. Money spent on subscribers' needs was seen as a "loss" to be minimized. The lower they kept that loss, the higher were their profits. Thinking in these terms means that companies have to find ways to reduce the amount spent on the people paying the premiums.

The companies argued that this was reducing waste and improving health care. I do not believe that. I feel that they go far beyond reducing waste and inefficiency and impair health care in the pursuit of profits, as I will argue in chapter 6.

As more and more employees were in effect forced into managed care contracts by employers who offered no alternatives, doctors who were not in the networks began to feel the pinch. They faced an inevitable choice: join or lose increasingly larger portions of their practices. Most doctors began to sign up with one and then many HMOs. HMO contracts do not prohibit doctors from joining as many other HMOs as they want.

Had all doctors refused to participate, as I and a few of my colleagues did and continue to do, managed care would have faded away.*

A revolution had occurred before anyone realized the full extent of the change. Managed care has helped in some ways and has hurt in many others. We will examine both and see if there is a positive cost-effectiveness ratio (to use one of their own favorite terms). Even more importantly, we will see what the *risk-benefit* ratio is, a much more important measure. In other words, are the benefits of managed care worth the risk they pose to your health? Are there ways to get those benefits without the risk?

Underlying all debates about health care are real issues that are seldom addressed directly. We will expose these issues here so that Americans can decide what they want for their own lives.

I believe that there are much better choices than managed care and government intervention. I will discuss in chapter 8 what I feel are better ways to achieve our health care goals.

NOTES

1. Doris Kearns Goodwin, *Lyndon Johnson and the American Dream* (New York: St. Martin's Press, 1991).

2. Laurie Zoloth-Dorfman and Suan Rubin, "The Patient as Commodity: Managed Care and the Questions of Ethics," *Journal of Clinical Ethics* 6 (Winter 1995): 339–57.

---

*I belong to no managed care in my private practice. I briefly signed on to two minor ones for research for this book, never saw any patients, and resigned after I had gathered the information I needed. I also spend some time in a nonprofit primary care clinic for a low-income population. The clinic participates in an HMO and I am in that plan for the clinic only. I am paid by the clinic and receive no money from the HMO.

3. Vote Smart: http://www.vote-smart.org/issues/Immigration/chap2/imm2b.htm, June 1998.

4. *White House Domestic Policy Council Health Security, The President's Report to the American People* (New York: Touchstone Books, Simon & Schuster, 1993), p. 8.

5. Milt Freudenheim, "Penny-Pinching H.M.O.'s Showed Their Generosity in Executive Paychecks," *Wall Street Journal*, April 11, 1995, D4.

6. Thomas Bodenheimer and Kip Sukkivan, "How Large Employers Are Shaping the Health Care Marketplace," *New England Journal of Medicine* 338 (April 2, 9, 1998): 1003–1007, 1084–87.

7. George Anders, *Health against Wealth, HMOs and the Breakdown of Medical Trust* (New York: Houghton Mifflin, 1996).

8. Ibid.

9. Nancy Ann Jeffrey, "Health-Care Costs Rise for Workers at Small Firms," *Wall Street Journal*, September 8, 1997, B2.

10. Robert Pear, "Health Spending Grew Slowly in '96 but Still $1 Trillion," *New York Times*, January 13, 1998, A15.

11. "Health Policies Don't Cover Many Expenses," *Wall Street Journal*, January 23, 1998, B7; "Out-of-Pocket Costs Are High, Study Shows," *UAARP Bulletin* 39 (April 1998): 7.

12. Anders, *Health against Wealth*.

13. Ibid.

14. Ibid., pp. 62–70.

5

Has Managed Care Succeeded? Slap! We Needed That. Or Did We?

Good has two meanings: it means that which is good absolutely and that which is good for somebody.

—Aristotle

In this chapter, we will begin to explore the validity of managed care's claims of success. In subsequent chapters, we will explore some of these issues in more depth and we will see how managed care inherently damages the doctor-patient relationship and interferes with the practice of good medicine as we defined it in chapter 2.

Some of the criticisms of the medical profession were correct. Some doctors had contributed to some of the problems health care faced.

Note the word *some.* Critics of the medical profession usually say, "doctors" did this or that, as if all 750,000 of them were one person. This kind of rhetorical generalization was effectively used to discredit the entire profession. It is akin to "all blacks are," "Jews always," and "Protestants never."

It is certainly true that there is some excess of treatment. This occurs for several reasons. First, it is profitable and some doctors succumb to the temptations. Secondly, defensive medicine stimulates unnecessary tests. Defensive medicine is the result of the rising threat of malpractice suits. Since doctors can be held accountable for omissions recognizable only in hindsight, they order more and more unnecessary tests in an attempt to cover all contingencies. Thirdly, the huge investment in test and treatment facilities provides a further economic incentive to do more rather than less.

Defensive medicine is a reality that must be addressed by reforming the way doctors are held accountable, which we will discuss in a later section on malpractice. Otherwise, it is a matter of character. Good doctors order what is right for patients; bad doctors order what is profitable for them. We cannot legislate or force doctors to be good. In attempting to do so, as managed care claims that it does, the cure is worse than the disease.

The majority of doctors in my experience order only the procedures they have carefully determined are right for each individual patient. Colleagues I work with always give me cogent, specific reasons for their actions, such as "Recent studies show" or "Usually we would do A but in this case this patient needs B because" or "I spent some time talking with Mr. Smith and considering his personality and lifestyle we should . . .". While it is true that I practice in a major city within the environment of a major medical center, I do not believe for one moment that we have a monopoly on goodness. There is a legion of good doctors throughout all communities who do what is right for their patients.

I believe that the profession would have come to reform itself. Even if that weren't true, even if the shock of managed care was necessary to shake the profession out of its traditional ways, the message has been heard loud and clear and it is time to move on.

New technology, although some of it costs much more, also has the potential to reduce costs more than any policy changes might. Many new surgical techniques simplify surgery, reduce time needed for recovery and improve results—all at a fraction of the cost. For example, orthopedic repair of knees once required hospitalization and major surgery that sliced open the whole knee. Now, with arthroscopic surgery that uses flexible fiberoptic instruments, the surgery is done through small incisions that leave the surrounding tissues intact, has better results, faster recovery, and reduces or eliminates hospital stays. Even knee replacement surgery, which requires major surgery, saves money because it spares patients from lives of expensive and unhappy disability in wheelchairs. Another example is the new understanding of the causes of heart disease. The use of cholesterol-lowering drugs, lifestyle changes, and earlier, more effective (and less expensive) treatment have combined to save more money in reduced heart disease than managed care ever could.

Managed care's pride and joy is that it supposedly ended health care inflation and brought runaway costs under control. "They saved us from terrible inflation," "they forced doctors to spend wisely," "they gave workers more money in their paychecks," and so on. I do not believe these claims are valid.

First, costs have not decreased. The only change has been that the rate of health care inflation has slowed. While that is good, in my review of the literature I have not seen any evidence that *proves* that managed care caused the slowing of inflation. Even if managed care could claim full credit for the slowing of health care cost inflation, I would still feel that the price we have paid has not been worth it. Since I feel that there are much better alternatives to managed care, such as those I offer in my last chapter, we do not have to suffer all the many problems of managed care to achieve our goals.

I believe that there is serious doubt that managed care brought about the reduction in health care expenditure growth. Much of it was due to Medicare and Medicaid cost-saving methods. Furthermore, we do not know what would have happened if managed care had not occurred. Inflation could have slowed for other reasons.

The claims for managed care's success in slowing the growth of medical costs are all based on the *assumption* that costs would have continued to increase without managed care's intervention. In real life, as opposed to an economist's graph of straight-line projections on paper, growth usually reaches a plateau and then levels off as the weight of the growth produces a braking effect. It seems much more plausible to me that that plateauing would have occurred without any artificial intervention because of the growing resistance to price increases and because the medical profession was beginning to heed the resistance and look for solutions.

We all make assumptions in everyday life because we have to act on the information available to us, even if incomplete. We look at what has happened and try to figure what will happen next. The natural guess or assumption would be that things will continue the way they have before.

Economists do the same thing and call them projections. Thus if a trend is increasing linearly, which means in a straight line on a graph, the projection would be that it will continue in a straight line, as is shown in figure 5.1. However, in social interactions and in biological mechanisms, things seldom continue in a straight line, because what occurs each day or at each step has a cumulative effect on what will happen next.

In real life, things develop much more often like the third graph in figure 5.1. In the previous chapter, we examined the plethora of rea-

FIGURE 5.1

Projection versus actual results

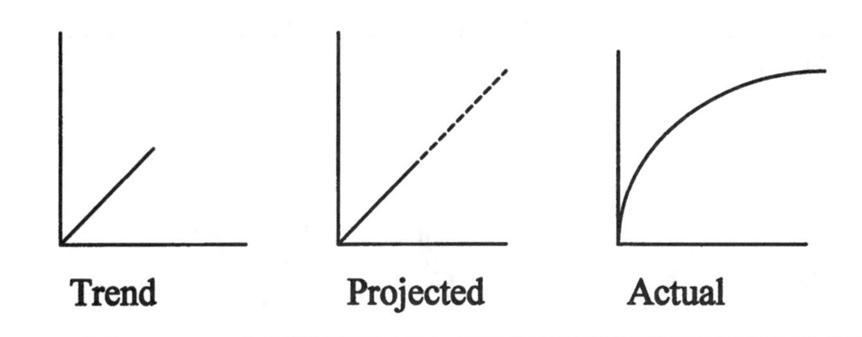

sons that have pushed total health care expenditures up. Some of these factors are tapering off or have exerted their full effect and will not increase further. Counterbalancing the continuing inflationary factors is the natural drag on growth and prices that occurs as buyers begin to resist, sellers feel the change in the market, and governments take action responding to political pressures.

There is another way to look at assumptions. Let us take an example where two events occur close together. It is easy to assume that they must be related as to cause and effect. A simple example involves the common cold, an upper respiratory infection due to a virus. Colds begin slowly, build to a peak and stay that way for a few days, then improve. There is no cure for the common cold, so that no treatment, not even antibiotics, makes any difference in the course of the disease. Colds are unpleasant and people think of antibiotics as wonder drugs that you just take and you will get better. It can be difficult to convince patients that anitbiotics are worthless for treating viruses.

In an attempt to convince patients with a little humor, we tell them that a cold lasts a week, but gets better in seven days if you take an antibiotic.

Suppose that a man takes an antibiotic at the beginning of a cold. when it is building up. Because the cold is in the worsening phase, he will get worse and think the antibiotic made him worse. If he takes it in the middle of the course of his virus, when it is in its plateau phase, he will just think it was worthless since he is getting no better. However, if he takes it just *before* the improvement begins, he will assume that the antibiotic cured him.

FIGURE 5.2

The arrow indicates an intervention in a process that builds up, plateaus, then improves.

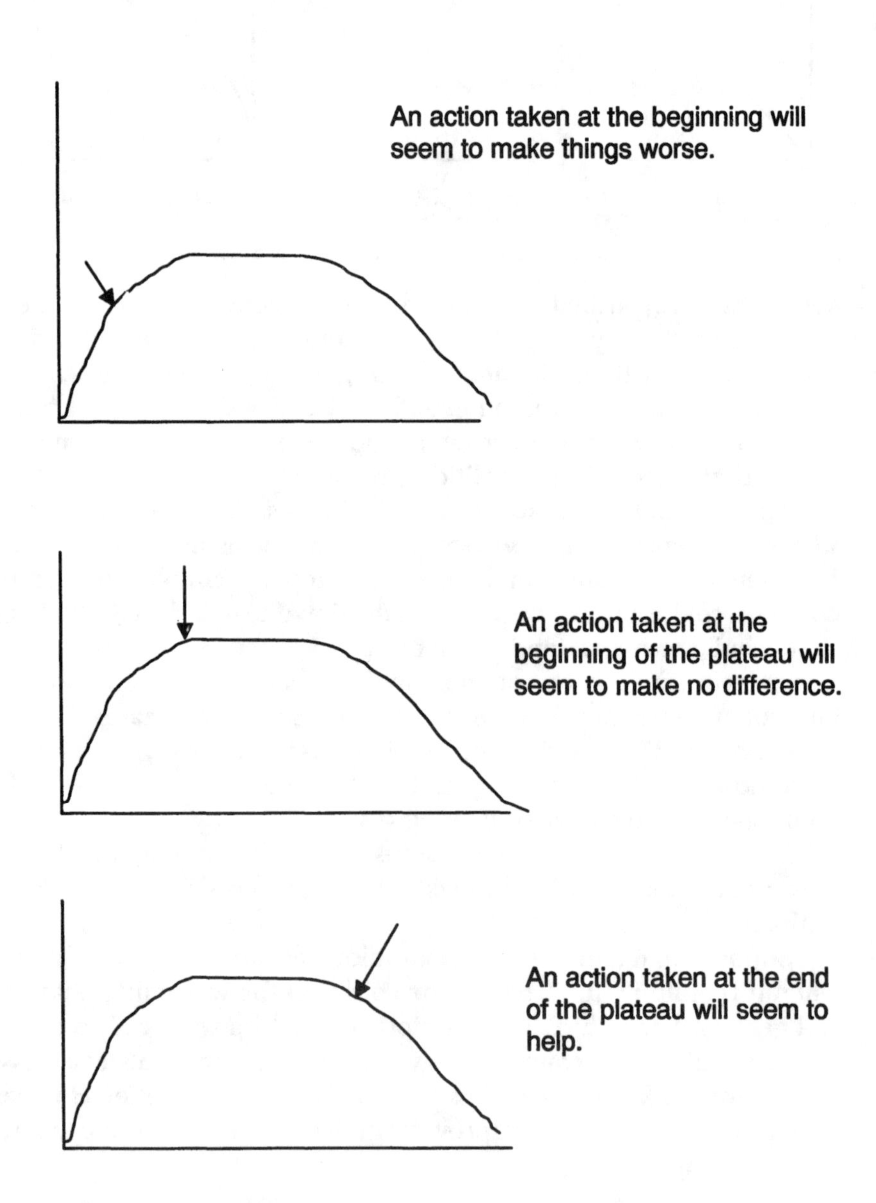

The three graphs in figure 5.2 illustrate these three scenarios.

Managed care came along at about the same time that health care inflation slowed, but the only proof that it was responsible are unproven assumptions that as we have seen are shaky at best.

The claim that managed care may have somewhat accelerated the rate at which obsolete and unnecessary procedures were eliminated may have some validity, but the effort to do so was well on its way before managed care, so it certainly does not deserve all the credit.

Managed care made some employers happy because the companies' premiums for health insurance for their employees stabilized, but the employees of those companies saw their own costs go up rapidly. While premiums may have stabilized for those employees who had to pay part of the premiums themselves, all patients under managed care saw an increase in what they had to pay out of pocket and a loss of benefits they used to have. Total health costs include premiums paid for insurance *plus* those expenses *not* covered by the insurance. We will discuss these changes in more detail in the next chapter. It is important to realize that managed care has forced a major shifting of the total cost for health care from employers to employees, even though the rate of increase in premiums has slowed.

One argument often made for reducing the increase in premiums is that companies will be able to pay higher salaries to employees, but there is no evidence that this happens. The bottom line and its effect on those wonderful stock options are much more enticing uses of savings than employees' paychecks. If companies want to pocket the savings for themselves, they should at least not promise otherwise.

One of the ignored hallmarks of the recent remarkable sustained economic boom is that the average person is benefiting far less than the upper managerial group. More people have jobs, but at lower pay, so they need two jobs to equal the buying power one used to provide.

Even if managed care resulted in a few hundred dollars more per year in employees' paychecks, that would hardly compensate for the much higher out-of-pocket medical costs and the denial of needed health care.

TO WHAT EXTENT HAS MANAGED CARE ACHIEVED ITS GOALS?

Managed care has brought modern business management techniques to health care. This is good for large enterprises, but I believe that a doctor's practice should be as a solo practitioner or as a member of a small group. Modern business methods have minimal value in those settings and may actually impair the delivery of care in some circumstances.

Managed care attempts to create incentives toward more prudent utilization of resources by rewarding doctors for doing less and by penalizing those who do not comply. This heavy-handed method pits the doctor's financial health against the patient's health needs in a way that never existed before. This is a perilous balance and there are much better and safer ways to achieve more sensible utilization in the proposal I make in the last chapter.

Under managed care, all patients are supposed to have a primary care doctor who coordinates their care and maintains continuity. This is a highly desirable goal, but one whose value is undercut by so many other aspects of managed care which we will examine in the following chapters, that the primary doctor has little time or incentive to perform the functions assigned.

Managed care *has* increased the performance of preventive efforts, one of its best accomplishments. This is laudable, but once again, I feel that this goal can be achieved equally well or better by other, better means.

Managed care has improved tracking of performance and outcomes in a few select areas. The most important outcomes, such as control of disease, improved management of illness, and so on, are not tracked. There is only one study that actually measured the care of seriously ill patients—managed care was significantly less successful for their patients than patients treated in traditional medical settings.[1] This is a powerful indictment of managed care. Health insurance's most important challenge is how it cares for you when you have a *serious* problem.

Managed care is of some temporary benefit to Medicaid patients. The federal government has allowed states to begin a trial of bringing some Medicaid patients under managed care. Under regular Medicaid, when the patients I see in the clinic need tests, consultations, or services outside of the clinic, it is extremely difficult to arrange what they need in a reasonable time or to get all the procedures they need, because the other facilities are so overloaded and there is so much turnover of their staff.

At present, when Medicaid patients are referred to other clinics, after very long waits for an appointment, they can be given short shrift or minimal care. Tests and treatments are dragged out over many weeks or months. If we request the outside clinic to move faster, the answer is to send the patients to the emergency room. Emergency rooms are intended for acute, serious illnesses, but they have become almost like a primary care doctor for many patients who have no insurance or Medicaid, since these patients know that the ER must treat them and charge them according to their ability to pay. ERs are not equipped, staffed, or intended for this purpose. Not matter how much the doctors and nurses want to help, they can give only limited, minimal care with little follow-up.

The delays and minimal care in ERs and overcrowded clinics are bad enough, but are particularly hazardous for this population, which is often in great need but very inexperienced in health care. They can be easily discouraged and do not know how to get what they require.

In contrast, when Medicaid patients come under a managed care contract, I can then refer them to participating private doctors, where they are seen more promptly and treated like other managed care patients.

Even though I will argue that managed care diminishes the quality of care for most patients, for the poor who have little or no care now, managed care is a least an improvement.

Unfortunately, the improved situation for the poor may be short lived. Since states and the federal government are cutting back on payments, the companies are discovering that it is not profitable enough for them. They are not used to having to pay for people who actually get sick and need care. Some companies are already beginning to withdraw from Medicaid contracts and undoubtedly more will follow.

The federal government is also providing incentives and new regulations to encourage managed care companies to offer products that are an alternative to traditional Medicare. The government pays the money to the managed care company and patients pay as they do now for Medicare. The Medicare HMOs add some benefits not available under regular Medicare, such as medication plans that require only a small copayment. I feel that these benefits will eventually be seen to be outweighed by the disadvantages, and as the government reduces payments, some of these added benefits are being withdrawn. Medicare HMOs are marketed directly to seniors and they started out well because they "cherry-picked" healthy patients. One cherry-picking recruiting tactic was to invite eligible seniors to dances and socials. Of course, only the healthy, active seniors could go. The recruiters somehow never got around to visiting nursing homes or homebound patients, the ones who would be likely to actually *need* care. Unfortunately for the companies, they are finding that even the seemingly healthy patients have greater needs than younger subscribers and that the plans are not as profitable as they had hoped. Companies are increasingly withdrawing from Medicare contracts as well.

Managed care's requirement to get approval for surgeries has been responsible for *some* reduction in unnecessary surgery, which has not only saved money, but even more importantly, spared patients procedures they did not need. However, as noted above, much of that reduction was about to happen anyway.

Newsweek columnist and economist Robert J. Samuelson said in a recent column that he very much dislikes his own managed care insurance, but that we need to put up with managed care because we need to control costs.[2] He claims that the good old days were not so good and by implication credits managed care with improving health care.

This claim of improved quality is a stretch, as I have been arguing. Samuelson quote from a new book called *Demanding Medical Excellence*, by Michael L. Millenson,[3] that criticizes bad medical practices over the past fifty years, such as unnecessary tonsillectomies and excessive bypass surgeries. The recognition and opposition to these practices came from within the medical profession, not insurance companies. Medicine is a highly dynamic field that questions its own ways and beliefs more than any other. There is room for great improvement, but medicine reexamines itself continuously and improves all the time. Pointing to the mistakes of the past does not prove that managed care is the answer.

Admissions to hospitals and the length of time patients stay in hospitals have been dramatically reduced, which is responsible for some of the control of health care expenses. Medicare began this trend and managed care accelerated it dramatically. Some of the savings were long overdue, but some amounted to cost shifting, which we will discuss in the next chapter.

Shorter stays are better for some patients, but the technique has become so extreme that many sick patients have to recover at home without needed assistance available only in a hospital. Mothers were forced to go home almost immediately after giving birth until state governments prohibited such rules. Women who underwent surgical removal of a breast for breast cancer were likewise forced home almost immediately, for which their term *drive-by mastectomies* was coined.

A recent article in the *Annals of Internal Medicine* cited a case of a woman with rapidly worsening severe angina.[4] She was rushed by helicopter from Nantucket Island to a major Boston hospital and underwent an emergency procedure to open her blocked artery. A stent (a wire mesh tube put inside an artery to keep it open) was placed. The procedure requires heparin (a drug that prevents clotting) infusions into a vein for a while to keep it open. The patient was then discharged after only *three* days, the insurance company's allowed length of stay for that procedure, with a needle and tube in place in her arm so she could give herself the heparin. The woman was first made to scramble, under duress, to find the money to *pay* for the heparin (she had no money with her since she was rushed by helicopter from her home). She was then sent to a friend's home in a cab in the middle of a blizzard. She finally arrived, but was so weak and exhausted that she barely made it into the house, only to suffer a recurrence of chest pain. Rushed back to the hospital, doctors found that the stent had clotted closed and the woman had suffered the heart attack that she had been flown to the great Boston hospital to prevent.

This is one of endless stories of patients sent home ill and weak to receive inferior care at home because someone decided that was the cost-effective way.

The rush to get patients out of the hospital quickly has had a major, deleterious effect on nursing homes and convalescent facilities. They are now servicing a much sicker population of patients, those who previously would have been brought to better condition by longer stays in the hospitals and rehabilitation. Rehabilitation is often severely limited under managed care. Many of these patients do far worse than they would have, since few nursing homes can provide what this sicker population requires.

One of the justifications for managed care is that it would create an incentive to use preventive measures to keep its customers healthy in order to improve its profits. Prevention was also an important emphsis of the HMO Act. Managed care companies strongly enforce certain standards, such as rates of immunizations, the use of cover sheets to help track and organize care, screening tests such as mammographies, and advice on prevention. These are important and beneficial practices. Unfortunately, managed care policies so overburden doctors and their staffs that they seldom have time or energy to effectively *accomplish* these mandates.

Prevention takes *time.* Manged care requires that doctors practice prevention, but they do not allocate the resources needed to accomplish it. That is hypocrisy of the worst order.

Managed care encourages the use of outpatient facilities to replace hospital care. That is a real benefit when procedures are minor and patients are healthy and at low risk for complications, but this has been so overdone that many patients are suffering.

Managed care companies carry out full credential checks on doctors who wish to contract with them to see their patients. This is a superficial screen, but at least it weeds out some egregiously bad applicants. HMOs reguarly review doctors' charts and hold them accountable for the quality of their records. Unfortunately, reviewing a written record does not guarantee that bad care will be detected or that good care will be adequately recognized.

There is one thing that some managed care companies are doing unusually well that would be harder to duplicate without the high profit flow they enjoy: innovative new outreach programs to service a long neglected need. A recent article describes three of these plans.[5] Nurses, social workers, and pharmacists visit homebound elderly and make frequent follow-up calls to pick up problems early, reduce isolation, and facilitate patients' compliance with complicated—or even simple—medical regimens. These patients need help in many aspects of their care, their lifestyle, their finances, their social contacts, and their living arrangements. Social service and visiting nurse services are enormously valuable assistance to patient care, but they are in short supply and those that exist are overloaded.

Large managed care capitation contracts* have the financial resources to provide this care. The doctors in these plans deserve full credit for providing such services and for bringing innovation and creativity to them. It would be harder to find financing for these services outside of managed care. Nursing and social worker services have been seen as too expensive up to now. Capitation groups see savings to their bottom line that more than justify the cost of the services. For example, identifying a patient's mistake in medication can save an expensive emergency room visit, and picking up a bronchitis early can save a later hospital admission for pneumonia. The doctors save money and the patients get better care.

These programs are not widespread and seem to be feasible only in large multimillion dollar capitation groups.

Managed care has introduced the *cost* of the care into the consciousness of medicine. It is certainly important that the profession be as prudent as possible in the use of limited resources. Managed care

---

*Captitation means that a group of doctors or individual doctors are given a set amount of money to care for a group of patients they are assigned. That is all they are paid no matter how much care is given those patients. Thus, there is a financial incentive to take care of those patients as inexpensively as possible and to keep them as healthy as possible. There is a strong incentive to do the least possible.

proponents claim that both quality and reasonable costs are accomplished, but I feel that cost has become the *only* real concern of managed care companies and that quality has suffered unacceptably. I believe that their pretentions to preserve and promote quality are unsuccessful at the least and have written this book to make my case.

In summary, managed care may have helped slow the growth of health care expenditures, modestly accelerated the trend toward more efficient care, encouraged some basic standards, temporarily upgraded care of some low-income patients, and made limited but important innovations in supportive services for homebound patients. I believe that both prior to managed care and currently there are much better ways to accomplish these goals, and without the very high price we pay for managed care that we shall see in the next chapter.

NOTES

1. John E. Ware Jr., et al., "Differences in 4-Year Health Outcomes for Elderly and Poor, Chronically Ill Patients Treated in HMO and Fee-for-Service Systems," *JAMA*, (October 2, 1996): 1039–47.
2. Robert J. Samuelson, "The Backlash against HMOs," *Newsweek* (March 9, 1998): 46.
3. Michael L. Millenson, *Demanding Medical Excellence* (Chicago: University of Chicago Press, 1997).
4. William G. Porter, "Venus on the Right," *Annals of Internal Medicine* 128 (March 15, 1998): 500–501.
5. Burt Schorr, "Giving Seniors Better Care without Burdening Doctors," *Physician's Management* (February 1998): 49–54.

6

What's Wrong with Managed Care and Government Control of Medicine?

It may be correct, but is it right?
—Saul Farber, M.D.

Public debates on health care are almost entirely on the level of strategy—how best to accomplish a goal. There has been very little debate on the goals themselves, the principles that underlie the issues, and the real implications they pose for our society.

There are serious moral, ethical, and societal issues that we need to resolve before any sensible decisions are made as to how to accomplish what we want as a country.

The first issue is how we preserve the freedom of all Americans to decide their own health care. The second is how we protect the doctor-patient relationship. The third is how we enhance physicians' ability to practice good medicine as I defined it in the chapter called "The Good Doctor." The fourth is how we protect the privacy of people when they seek medical care. The fifth is how we maintain the quality of care provided by physicians and the other health professions. Sixth is how we respect the rights of physicians and nurses to practice ethical medicine that is professionally satisfying and financially rewarding commensurate with the value and difficulty of what they do. Seventh is how we hold medical professionals accountable for their performance in a reasonable and productive way. Eighth is how we fairly and effectively allocate limited resources when need outstrips supply. Ninth is how we deal compassionately and helpfully with those who are chronically ill, disabled, terminally ill, or otherwise dependent on the the kindness and help of others. Tenth is how we prevent as many problems as we can and how we improve the fitness level of the population. Eleventh is how we serve the needs of the poor, the homeless, and others who are financially unable to compete for health care resourses. Twelfth is how we protect and enhance our most precious members of society, our children. And last, but certainly not least, is how much of our economic resources do we devote to achieving all of these goals.

In this chapter and in those that follow, I will give my personal views as a practicing physician directly responsible for the care of patients. I have treated thousands of patients face-to-face over the past thirty-four years and I express what I know to be the needs and rights of people when they seek help. To reiterate what I said at the beginning, I will attempt in this book to be the representative for patients and their doctors.

First we will examine in some detail how I feel managed care and government-run medical care adversely affect good medical care. Then we will explore some additional important issues. In the last chapter I will outline why and how I would radically change the way we currently administer health care.

Please note that nowhere do I imply that managed care is in any way illegal. There have been some serious cases of mismanagement and fraud by some managed care companies and some managed care executives. This book does not concern itself with those who violate the law or mismanage their corporation. What we are concerned with here is whether the process of managed care and government-run care, when performed legally and effectively, is the best way for us to provide health care in this country.

I believe that there are many things that both managed care corproations and the government do that are correct but are not right. That is, their actions are legal and feasible but far from the proper way to do things.

What follows next is a series of problems as I see them.

HMOs SAY THEY MANAGE CARE, BUT THEY REALLY MANAGE MAINLY COST

As we noted earlier, Paul Ellwood and others had envisioned HMOs as a way to stimulate interest in better and more efficient care by creating good-spirited competition. Ellwood foresaw research on how to improve quality and outcomes and how to find ways to use valuable limited resources more productively. In a world where the best possible outcome for all is sought, this may well have worked. But ours is a competitive, entrepreneurial world. The nature of business is to use limited resources to achieve the greatest return on investment at the least cost. Sale price is limited by the marketplace, so cost is the key to profit. And managed care, while being focused on health care delivery, is also (some would say first and foremost) a business.

Business had previously never succeeded in the health care world because in that world cost was never allowed to be the issue. What matters is helping people, saving lives, finding cures. Over the past thirty years, I have seen countless managers of clinics and hospitals arrive full of confidence, only to slink away with their tails between their legs. But that changed, of course, when the managed care executives arrived on the scene.

When quality of care is placed above cost, options to save money are more limited. Theoretically, one should be able to achieve both, but in the real world, when profit becomes important, cost factors end up outweighing concerns about quality health care. Managing costs, maximizing profits, and even a bit of reasonable greed (as a compelling motive for success) are appropriate for business. The point of business is increasing sales and profits by reducing expenses in ways that are legal, ethical, and permit you to sell your product. Such a view has been considered good for centuries and is part of the reason we are such a successful country. Capitalism, within reasonable limits, is without a doubt the best economic system available compared to the less desirable alternatives.

But we must ask ourselves: should the delivery of our health care be a business, a commodity to be sold like clothing or furniture? If you buy a bad shoe or a non–New York bagel, you may choose just to throw it away and buy a better one next time. All you have lost is time and a little money. Good health is infinitely more important than any product you can purchase. Disease and disability impair or destroy nearly everything else in your life. If your car wears out, you can always get another, but you only have one body. Replacement parts are very hard to find, very expensive, painful to install, and seldom work as well as your original equipment.

Good business practice does not leverage (borrow against) the company more than it can afford to lose or pay for. A person should not leverage his or her body at all, because no part is expendable or worth the risk. **You must decide whether society should allow others to gamble with your health for their purposes.**

Whatever the original intention, managed care as a corporate enterprise is now driven only by cost. A surgeon at NYU recently had to get approval for a surgery, so he spoke to a medical director. The director, a managed care doctor, said, "Don't you remember me? I was one of your students." She then went on to tell him some of the inside methods in their company. Most striking was that she earned 10 percent of the cost of all care that she *denied*.[1] In other words, if she said that a procedure worth five hundred dollars, could not be performed, then she earned a fee of fifty dollars for saving the managed care facility the expense of the procedure. Talk about incentive! That is an incentive to save only money, not lives.

A far more detailed account of managed care methods is in an astounding article in the March 9, 1998, *U.S. News & World Report*.[2] Linda Peeno, M.D. was a medical director for several managed care companies over a four-year period. Her article is required reading for anyone who wishes to understand this new corporate medical phenomenon. She describes the pressures from her bosses and coworkers to save money at any cost. An anonymous note Peeno once found on a case file said, "Approve this, and it will be your last!" Limiting and denying services were the medical director's job, and she was repeatedly warned that she would be fired if she were not strict enough.

"I couldn't overcome the pressures to deny care, to manipulate medical guidelines and contract language, and to push physicians toward some practices that endangered patient care. I was surprised to find that it made little difference whether the company was for-profit or not-for-profit. The basics of managed care were the same."[3]

She describes the team-player pressures that compelled all the employees to save money for the company under the rationale that this was somehow good for the country. "No one dared think, much less ask, what gave us the right to sacrifice the well-being, and even life, of particular individuals for this so-called good."[4]

Managed care providers now routinely deny admission to the hospital the night before surgery, insisting that patients come in the same day of the operation. They also dictate what hospital should be used for the surgery, even if it is much farther away than more convenient local facilities.

A doctor requested that Peeno grant an exception for an ill eighty-year-old man who needed bowel surgery and would find it very difficult to handle the intensive laxatives needed to clean out his bowel for surgery. "Without this pre-op admission, this frail man would have to drive himself to the hospital [sixty miles away] almost in the middle of the night, after hours of laxatives and withholding of fluids. When I approved the request, I got a call from my physician supervisor, angrily telling me that we did not pay for creature comforts!"[5] If they consider it to be a "creature comfort" for an eighty-year-old man, imagine what they would want *you* to endure.

Peeno notes that managed care tracks many things that relate to cutting costs, but the one thing it does not track is the health outcome of its denials and limitations of services. Apparently, that would make its self-serving rationalizations too difficult, even for those who run the HMOs.

Dr. Peeno quit her managed care job and is now head of her hospital's ethics committee and is a nationally recognized expert on the problems of managed care.

MANAGED CARE DOES NOT REDUCE COSTS, IT ONLY REDUCES CARE

In the same issue of *U.S. News & World Report,* a senior editor writes that, in effect, managed care is a necessary evil (my expression, not hers, but it represents the gist of the article) because it was so important to reduce costs.[6] *Newsweek*'s Robert Samuelson expressed the same sentiment in the article described in the last chapter.[7]

I cannot agree with them. I believe that managed care has not really reduced costs, nor was managed care necessary to achieve the goal of more efficient health care. What managed care did do was reduce the amount of health care delivered to subscribers, in effect reducing the amount of product being offered to the public. The cost of health care only leveled off; it did *not* decline. Even leveling off is a major improvement, but, even if managed care deserves credit, I believe it has come at far too high a price.

Demand for health care continued to grow under managed care since people did not stop getting sick, but the supply was reduced by managed care by reducing the amount and type of care that would be paid for. Increased demand and reduced supply usually cause prices to rise, but, in this case they did not because prices were artificially controlled by the managed care contracts. The health care segment of the economy is so large and complex that it is unlikely we will ever be able to estimate the full effect of managed care on prices and expenditures. Managed care claimed such success in controlling prices and costs that it makes one wonder why expenditures and prices merely slowed in growth rather than actually declining below the levels before managed care took hold of the bulk of health care insurance.

I believe part of the problem is that managed care imposes a considerable amount of overhead. It siphons off up to 30 percent or more of the premiums paid by subscribers[8] and uses that money for its own profit and to pay for the huge executive salaries and high administrative overhead it needs to enforce its policies. It is my impression that health care has been so decimated that health costs of this country might have even declined had managed care not siphoned off so many billions of dollars. From 1960 to 1990, the country went through enormous changes that forced health care costs up very rapidly, as I outlined in chapter 4. The inflationary impact of those factors had played out by 1990, and we were probably in for a period of relative stability. (In the first decades of the twenty-first century, the further aging of the baby boom generation and the impact of AIDS will cause another major inflationary increase, and other yet unanticipated factors may contribute as well.) Therefore, if costs were cut, the total health care expenditures should have gone down. They have not.

Let me give just a few examples of how some costs have been cut. A colleague who is one of the top general surgeons at my medical center told me his fees have been cut by 50 to 75 percent, and they continue to go down by 20 percent per year. A specialist in internal medicine told me that a visit for which he charged one hundred dollars ten years ago would today be reimbursed only twenty dollars under a managed care contract.

Statistically, doctors' incomes have increased. These surveys are conducted by the American Medical Association, which certainly has a vested interested in accurate results. However, no matter how carefully the survey is conducted, I believe that it is inevitably skewed because I believe the survey reaches a disproportionate percentage of the most successful doctors, so that it represents the income of only the more fortunate members of the profession. What cannot be well reflected in those figures are the incomes of those doctors who do not participate in any managed care or who do but continue to spend time with patients and do not increase their patient volume to compensate for the lower payments per patient. These are doctors who refuse to compromise their care for the sake of their incomes, but they are paying a high price. As I mentioned previously, many doctors do not even have the option of resisting the penetration of managed care into their practices, and few can afford drastic reductions in their income.

A colleague of mine is a gastroenterologist, which means he specializes in the care of diseases of the digestive organs. He has two young children. So many of his patients came under managed care that he had to sign up with many managed care companies or close his practice. He told me that he is making half as much money and working twice as long, with quadruple the frustration. He works until twelve each night and has loads of paperwork to do at home. He is torn between spending time with his family and maintaining an income to provide for them.

Doctors who decline to participate in managed care eventually suffer the greatest loss. So few patients have traditional insurance today that the pool of available non–managed care patients has shrunk to levels that support very few practices. A clear conscience does not put bread on the table.

There are cost reductions forced upon every segment of health care. Where is all that money going? It is not hard to find. It went into the pockets of corporations which reaped billions of dollars in health care premiums savings by joining HMOs, or which shifted the burden of additional premiums and copays to their employees. The other beneficiaries were the managed care companies which helped these large businesses. Investors who were smart enough to buy stock in corporations in the managed care business during the early years reaped a windfall.

Until recently, managed care companies had billion-dollar cash reserves—money they had earned but not spent. George Anders reported their excesses.[9] In 1994, for example, ten companies together had *$10.5 billion* dollars in liquid assets; United Healthcare alone had $2.6 billion. This far exceeded what the insurance companies needed in back-up reserves which insurance companies are required to maintain to cover heavy losses. Money poured in faster than they knew how to spend it. Their executives routinely took home multimillion dollar compensation packages. Even now, when some of the companies are not doing as well, the executives continue to make huge salaries.

I firmly believe that health care costs would likely have flattened out on their own at the time that managed care was taking over the market. The companies have taken credit for a trend that was already underway, and they have gutted the health care system for their own profit. The savings achieved have gone mostly to them, with only small savings and reduced quality of care for patients.

Cost shifting occurs in other ways as well. Cost shifting means that one entity reduces its costs by having another entity take on the burden. A typical managed care premium for a family in New York in a group of at least two employees is in the range of $7,000 to $8,000 per year. The same policy for a group of one or for an individual family buyer is in the range of $12,000 to $17,000! The difference of one family or person *versus* a "group" of two means double the cost. (The insurance companies claim that single family or single person buyers tend to have more health care expenses than people in groups. Beware of such convenient self-serving industry claims.)

The intent of the Kennedy-Kassebaum bill, which became law in 1996 as the Health Care Portability and Accountability Act, a law that had attempted to ensure that if employees lost their jobs or switched jobs they would not lose their health insurance, has been completely thwarted. The law sets no restriction on the *cost* of the continued insurance and the companies have gleefully charged those high individual rates. How many people can afford to keep up insurance that suddenly costs twice as much?

U.S. News & World Report claimed that one of managed care's benefits is that it allows more employers to offer health insurance.[10] If only this were true. First, instead of using health care insurance as a beneift to its entire employment, one of the major trends has been to fire employees, then rehire them as temporary workers *without* health insurance. Second, the lower premiums are possible only because there is less care given, so that the people who do have coverage receive much less benefit from it. In the early days of managed care, sicker people were pushed out of managed care and into high-cost individual insurance or into the ranks of the uninsured. Their policies were canceled for obscure reasons, or there were so many denials of care that the policyholders gave up.

Charging more for less healthy people, individuals, and the self-employed permits the reduced rates for employees. This involves a very practical philosophical issue: how we allocate risk and who pays for it. We will discuss this at length in the "Issues" chapter (12).

Another important type of cost-shifting is the fact that, as managed care restricts tests, consults, and other services, patients who need them anyway must pay for them out of their own pockets. This cost-shifting—from the insurer to the patient—allows the managed care company to charge lower premiums. This obscures the fact that total cost to the patient (premiums plus out-of-pocket) is the same or higher than under traditional, fee-for-service indemnity insurance! This has been studied and reported in many ways, for example as in a Congressional Budget Office study.[11] Whatever proportion of the premium is paid by employer and subscriber, the cost shift is the same.

Thus, there has been considerable *shifting* that masquerades as reduction: costs shifted to smaller, vulnerable segments of the population, income shifted out of doctors' and others' pockets, and enormous profits shifted into the hands of large corporations and a tiny handful of very hungry entrepreneurs.

MANAGED CARE SO REDUCES THE TIME DOCTORS CAN SPEND WITH THEIR PATIENTS THAT THE QUALITY OF CARE IS SEVERELY IMPAIRED

Perhaps the saddest loss in today's health care system is time. Managed care has stolen the time you should have with your doctor. The doctor who is paid less than 20 percent of what was previously paid for a patient visit will have to see *six to seven times* the number of patients in the same amount of time to even try to maintain an income. The fees were reduced by as much as 80 percent and doctors' administrative costs were increased significantly, mainly by need for more employees to handle the paperwork and approval calls. The result is that the doctor has very little time with each patient. The effect of patient overload is magnified because it requires a much higher overhead to see a high volume of patients, including often two or more additional secretaries to handle the managed care paperwork. A major portion of the doctor's and staff's time and energy is now spent on complying with all the rules and regulations of the managed care companies, administration, and fighting with them to win approval for treatments for patients.

Managed care forces doctors to work many more hours. It is as if my friend the gastroenterologist's young children have had their father stolen from them. A recent article in the *Annals of Internal Medicine* discusses the impact of doctors' long hours on their children.[12] One doctor's child said she had no memory of her father before she was eight years old because she was never able to stay up late enough to see him before that age. A four-year-old asked his mother, "Did Daddy die?"

A good doctor spends time to listen to, examine, and counsel patients. Every characteristic of good care takes time. *Stealing time steals good care.*

Even if there are attempts to improve managed care, Medicare, Medicaid, and any other kind of insurance plan, if they continue to underpay for time, quality will be lost.

I believe that an internist or famly physician cannot provide high quality care for the thirty to forty patients per day that are the standard of "productivity" today. "Productivity" is the managed care term that refers to how many patients the doctor sees each day. It means either see thirty to forty or more patients per day or we do not want you. I have checked dozens of managed care–dependent job offers all over the country and the job requirements are the same.

To me, ten to twelve patients a day is a very busy day and I prefer less. Most of the general internists I know and respect who are not in managed care all concur with this figure. In other specialties such as obstetrics or dermatology, patients come for limited, specific problems, and many visits are for brief follow-ups, so specialists like these can see more patients per day and still treat them fairly.

A young internist recently told me how he had organized a large group of fellow internists and obtained large, profitable managed care contracts. He claimed that he could see up to forty patients per day and still spend enough time with them by working nonstop twelve-hour days and being "very efficient." That means he also has to take and make large numbers of telephone calls and at least some hospital visits. He says his managed care contracts have boosted his income.

Let's give him the benefit of the doubt and assume that he is able to accomplish the feat of spending time and giving good care to so many patients in one day. It leaves open the question of finding time to research care for those hundreds of patients he sees and keeping up to date on internal medicine. But even if he is the superman he claims, he admitted that after only a few years he is already getting burned out and cannot keep it up. He said he would soon be hiring a physician's assistant, which will place an additional barrier between him and his patients and reduce the time he spends with them.

Another doctor I interviewed loves managed care because he never spent much time with patients anyway. He also claimed to be very efficient and said he could quickly size up a patient's problem and decide treatment swiftly. I asked him what he would do if the patient had more questions or more than one problem and whether he did any preventive care. He said he would have the patient come back for separate visits for each complaint. I do not believe that it is satisfactory to fragment care in that way, nor do I think it is fair to make patients visit frequently just for the doctor's financial benefit.

The increased patient load has had a huge impact on psychiatry, in which visits are sometimes down to as little as *eight minutes.*[13] One doctor recalled a patient who came in and asked if she could get a drink of water; she was anxious and her mouth was dry. He had to tell her that she could, but, since the fountain was down the hall, it would exhaust her session time. If a new merger goes through, Magellan Health Services, which already controls 90 percent of the country's psychiatric hospitals and two behavioral care companies, would then control the mental health care of fifty million people![14]

James Wrich, head of a company that consults for HMOs, estimates that HMOs have scaled back psychiatric services by up to 60 percent. He estimates that "today, untreated psychiatric problems cost $435 billion, or 40 percent of the nation's entire $1.1 trillion health-care budget."[15]

Psychiatric care was limited under traditional insurance and the number of subscribers with mental health benefits has increased under managed care. This seems to be an advantage for managed care except that the funding for mental health visits is so limited that it is of very questionable value. Psychiatric problems are every bit as real and as important as any physical problem, yet they have been terribly neglected both in the past and under managed care. The cost in human misery, lost productivity, and secondary damage to the lives of families, friends, and coworkers is immeasurable.

There is also a continuing prejudice against mental problems. The first thing I have to do when broaching the subject with patients is to help them see that there is no stigma attached to seeking help and they will not lose themselves in some arcane process. We are body *and* mind. Until we fully recognize the importance of both, we will be short-changing ourselves dangerously.

The return on investment of solving these mental health problems exceeds anything in business or finance. What hampers funding is the sense that treatments go on forever. Modern psychiatry is result-oriented, seeking briefer but effective ways to restore patients to full function and enjoyment of life. This requires more than a few minutes, however, despite what managed care would like. Managed care has encouraged the use of drug treatment over therapy since even expensive drugs are cheaper than therapy sessions. But drugs alone, however, solve few problems.

Internists must equally attend to both the bodies and the minds of their patients. Consider the examples I gave in the "Good Doctor" chapter (2) of the patients whose emotional states so affected their physical health. It took hours and many visits, listening and winning their confidence, before they were able to share such private problems. How will that happen in a patient-a-minute world?

A wealthy foreign patient flies to New York to see me for her medical care. In her country, there were so few doctors that although she was extremely rich and knew the doctors from her university days, she was nevertheless badly mistreated, to the point that she might have died had we not corrected her treatment. She said that, at home, a single doctor had so many patients (because there are too few doctors) that he would ask her a question, but, while she would be considering her answer, the doctor would be turning to the next patient. Is that what we want for America?

Speed-medicine breeds error. With no time for listening and counseling, zero room for reflection and review, doctors will make many more mistakes in diagnostics, prescriptions, and procedures, and patients will be far less equipped to follow instructions properly. Many doctors have admitted to me that this is the case, but they feel powerless to do anything about it.

Some doctors argue that when they see large numbers of patients, many are there just for colds, quick follow-ups, and the like. The time saved on these brief visits can be used for those who need more care. Yet that means those short visits cannot be an opportunity to reach out to the patient, to encourage more exercise or dietary control, and to see how things are going at home.

Patients often come for one thing, but then use the opportunity to ask about something else that is important to them. Patients might think they have a minor problem but when it turns out to be something serious that needs an extended visit, what happens to that efficient schedule? Are you going to tell a dying patient to come back next week?

In most cases, it's not the doctor's choice to practice such high patient volume. It's not merely necessary to maintain a reasonable income; their employers require it! Doctors may be summarily expelled if they fail to meet specific quotas.

It is simply impractical to think that such a system is a substitute for good care as I have defined it. A high-volume system can provide only barely adequate care and only under certain circumstances. In fact, private communications from malpractice lawyers reveal their absolute delight with managed care. They predict an epidemic rise in malpractice cases against doctors and whisper that there are already many in the pipeline. The rush to diagnose and go on to the next patient inevitably leads to missed symptoms or other errors and oversights. As we will discuss at length later in this chapter, mananged care-companies are essentially immune from being held liable for their doctors' actions.

When I was studying patterns of medical care in clinics, I worked briefly in different clinics under the high-volume conditions characteristic of most such facilities. As a very experienced physician, I could zero in on the immediate problem and apply necessary care effectively and quickly, but there was no time for anything else. When I did spend extra time with a patient, I was quickly chastised. However, I can testify to the strain such volume and intensity produced in the short periods I was there, so I can see how the managed care internist could burn out.

I do not like to practice medicine only for affluent patients, yet I refuse to participate in assembly-line medicine. Fortunately, I was able to find a well-funded primary care clinic where I see patients a few days per week. We average one half-hour per patient. That is not quite as much time as I have available in my private office, but it allows reasonably good care of patients and many times better than what they usually receive.

New York State standards mandate that physicians go beyond the bare minimum necessary for the acute problem the patient has come for, yet the bare minimum is the only way to cope with high-volume situations. Managed care claims to maintain even higher standards, requiring all kinds of counseling and preventive care, *but it refuses to pay for compliance with its own standards by paying doctors too little to spend the time required.*[16] **Setting meaningless standards whose only purpose is marketing and legal compliance is dishonest and abusive.**

The lack of time with patients inherent in the profit motive of managed care and the cost-cutting of nonprofit and government health care systems is the hidden but major detrimental cost of alleged health care "reform." I wonder if we can survive being reformed.

THE DOCTOR–PATIENT RELATIONSHIP IS SUFFERING UNDER MANAGED CARE AND GOVERNMENT CARE

As I said at the beginning of this book the doctor-patient relationship *is* medicine. Sir William Osler, one of the great teachers and innovators who helped establish modern medicine, also helped revolutionize medical education. Before Osler, medical students were taught from books and rarely saw actual patients until they went out into the world to practice on their own.

Osler said that to study medicine without books was to sail an uncharted sea, but to study medicine without patients was to never set sail at all. Osler took his students to the patient's bedside, interviewed the patient in front of the students, and correlated that with the science they were learning. He was renowned for his ability to learn about his patients and to form a warm bond with them.

While I was in medical school at the Columbia University College of Physicians and Surgeons, the school was celebrating its bicentennial. We learned in an atmosphere steeped in traditions inspired by Oslerian-type principles. We were taught to listen to patients and to respect them as people.

I recently spoke with Dr. Michael Cohen, my first clinical supervisor in medical school when I was a third-year student. Then and now he combines a brilliant mind, a deep knowledge of medicine, and the highest standards of ethical and caring medicine. Cohen said that, in his opinion, the whole *raison d'être* of managed care is completely contrary to that of quality medical care.

Great medicine is about people, not diseases. In contemporary medicine, the vital link between the patient and the doctor is being destroyed. We discussed this at some length earlier. Now we will examine more specifically how managed care and government health care programs have interfered.

The theft of time just described is the first step. The next is that the insurance programs become competitors for your doctor's loyalty by the incentives that they offer, by the virtual fee-splitting that occurs, and by the adversarial relationships they create, as we shall see in the next chapter.

NOTES

1. Personal communication, anonymous by request.
2. Linda Peeno, "What is the Value of a Voice?" *U.S. News & World Report* (March 9, 1998): 40–46.
3. Ibid.
4. Ibid.
5. Ibid.
6. Susan Brink, "HMOs Were the Right Rx," *U.S. News & World Report* (March 9, 1998): 47–50.
7. Robert J. Samuelson, "The Backlash against HMOs," *Newsweek* (March 9, 1998): 46.
8. George Anders, *Health against Wealth, HMOs and the Breakdown of Medical Trust* (New York: Houghton Mifflin, 1996).
9. Ibid.
10. Brink, "HMOs Were the Right Rx."
11. Physicians Who Care, "Managed Care Does Not Reduce the Growth of Health Care Expenses," http://pwc.org/ganske/growth.htmls/25/98.

12. Lawrence J. Hergott, "The Time of Three Dynasties: Reflections on Imbalance in the Practice of Medicine," *Annals of Internal Medicine* 128 (January 15, 1998): 149–51.

13. Katherin Eban Finkelstein, "The Sick Business," *The New Republic* (December 29, 1997): 23–27.

14. Ibid., p. 25.

15. Ibid.

16. Jennifer Fisher Wilson, "Doctors Caught in Prevention Squeeze," *ACP Observer* 18 (February 1998): 1.

7

More Ways in Which Managed Care Impairs Your Relationship with Your Doctor

WHAT HAPPENS WHEN DOCTORS MUST SERVE MANY MASTERS

We discussed previously that a good physician should serve only the patient who has sought the doctor's services. There must be no dual allegiance. In your daily life, you consider the motives of other people. Are they acting on your behalf, on their own, or for someone else? You judge your sources all the time. Is the information you are hearing for your benefit or the benefit of person selling you something? You enter an appliance store to buy a clothes dryer. The salesperson shows you an expensive model although you said you just wanted a simple machine. Is he pushing the expensive one because he gets a commission or because the sales manager told the sales crew they had to meet a quota of high-priced units? You find termites in your house. You secure estimates from five different companies—the prices vary widely. You go back to the more expensive one and tell him the lowest competitive price; his price comes down. Then you find one company that shows you how *no* treatment is needed. Were the others serving you or themselves only? Finally, a computer program is $29.95 at one computer chain store and the exact same program is $49.95 at another store. You wonder if one has too many in inventory or the other thinks it is a hot program. As these examples show, we constantly have to judge the validity of the advice we are given. We weigh what we know about the product, what motives contribute to the advisor's decision, and then we judge the reliability of the source. For example, we might believe the termite man who recommended no treatment because that advice is against his own self-interest and thus more likely to be in our interest.

With medical treatment, it is harder to shop around and more difficult for the public to try to learn about the "product." The news media feature daily stories on medical news, but a significant percentage is wrong or misleading. There are books for laypersons and, now, an enormous amount of material on the Internet. Unfortunately, much of the material is wrong and much of it is motivated by self-interest (such as unproven claims for herbal remedies) or well-intentioned people caught up in their enthusiasm for their cause. It is very hard for a layperson to make sense of it all. In addition, a little information can be worse than none at all. Even accurate information can be misleading if acted upon without understanding the context and without the appropriate training. Chest pain with pain down the left arm frightens everyone, but a doctor knows a dozen alternative explanations besides the heart attack most people would fear, and many of the alternatives are quite innocuous.

Evaluating services is very different because each depends on the quality and skill of the people who perform them. We hired a plumber for a job; he did it so badly that it resulted in months of problems. On another job, a higher priced plumber did it properly the first time. The more expensive one was the far better deal. The same principle holds true in medicine, but the consequences can be far more dire than pipes that repeatedly back up or a basement that is flooded.

In the past, people usually knew their doctors, who were their neighbors or members of their communities. The public had a pretty good idea of what kind of person the doctor was and they had faith in the professionalism that marked the practice of medicine. There was an unspoken but powerful covenant between the doctor and the patient: It was understood that the doctor put the needs of the patient above all else. Today, when a doctor recommends a treatment, you have to worry if the doctor is motivated by the *patient's* best interest, the doctor's own income, the necessity of pleasing a managed care company, or the concern about malpractice claims.

The managed care executive I referred to at the beginning of this book said that there were only three incentives for doctors: (a) fee-for service, which is an incentive to do too much; (b) capitation, which is an incentive to do too little; or (c) salary, which is an incentive to go home at five o'clock. This man does not deserve the title "doctor" because he seems to have forgotten the motives of a true professional: to serve the patient, to keep one's skills and knowledge at the highest level, to give fully of one's time and effort, to care about one's patients as if they were one's own family, to be the best doctor one can be, to live up to the spirit of the Hippocratic Oath that every doctor swears to at graduation!

Managed care is battering down the professionalism of today's physicians. Many doctors still resist, but they are human. They have families to support and their options have been taken from them.

Managed care companies are now in complete control. They set the fees and capitation allowances so the doctor has little leeway. He is paid the same whether he treats a problem by telephone in five minutes or spends two hours with one patient in the office. The financial restrictions are so great that he can no longer afford to spend two hours with a patient, or seldom even more than fifteen minutes, regardless of the person's need.

In some plans the doctor's contract includes a "withhold," which means that some percentage, often 20 percent, of the money owed the doctor is *retained* by the insurance company. Sometime around six months after the year is over, the insurance company calculates whether the doctors spent more or less money than the company wanted. If they had not ordered too many tests and consults, then the insurance company will give them the money they earned eighteen months before. However, if they have not met expectations, then the insurance company keeps the withheld money the doctors earned.

This shifts some of the financial risk from the insurer to the doctors, but the insurer retains total administrative control and their own profits are preserved. This increased financial risk, along with the calls, denials, and other control mechanisms the insurer uses, puts enormous pressure on the doctors to conform to the insurer's requirements even if they are contrary to what the doctors feel is best for the patient.

If a doctor has ordered more tests or consults than the company likes, the doctor gets a call from the medical director. "Dr. Jones, I see that you've ordered thirty-five chest X-rays in the past six months. Most of our doctors order fewer than fifteen. Do you really need all those X-rays?" If Dr. Jones's numbers do not improve, he will get a letter that says that there are too many doctors on the panel and that his services are no longer needed. He will have to find a new source of patients, which is difficult and is a severe economic blow. His ex-patients, who had finally gotten to know him a little, and he them, will have to start all over again with another doctor.

It is vitally important that the only person the doctor works for is *you.* As we defined before, all managed care, in all its many forms and varieties, is direct service insurance. The insurance company employs the doctor, the hospital, and the ancillary services. You pay the insurance company to use those services.

When you deal with an independent doctor, you are the only employer and you can directly judge the motives and quality behind the service and advice. When some other entity is pulling the strings, you are dealing with a distant, faceless presence that is deciding your fate.

Medicare and Medicaid technically are indemnity insurers, in that they reimburse for bills and the doctors and others do not work for them. In effect, however, they are as controlling as managed care. They set the rules and the fees by law and there are stiff penalties for noncompliance.

Patients can decide well enough if they trust the doctor they see before them, but how do they judge a faceless, distant bureaucracy whose actions are behind the scenes and whose motives are cost control and profit?

HOW MANAGED CARE DENIES CARE AGAINST THE DOCTOR'S JUDGMENT

Under managed care, doctors must get prior approval from the company for many tests and procedures. If approval is denied, the company will not pay for the service. Sometimes, the doctor is told over the telephone that the service is approved, but after the service is provided to the patient, the company can rescind the approval and refuse to pay. Their rationale is that phone approvals are provisional. The doctor and patient have no way to resolve the uncertainty beforehand. If a service is denied and all appeals fail, the patient can then either pay for it or do without. Managed care contracts include some right of appeal, but, with few exceptions, the appeal is only to a higher level in the company. There has been some move to involve outside arbitration services and some recent court rulings, but in general, the odds are stacked against the doctor and patient.

Some routine care is approved, though often only after a struggle or with some concession, and some is denied even though the expense is modest. Many expensive and controversial items do not fare as well. The more expensive the procedure, the more opposition it will engender, as Linda Peeno revealed in the article discussed previously.

Many critics agree that the denials are clearly arbitrary and unfair. Peeno was put under tremendous pressure to deny expensive care in any way she could, regardless of need. Recall also the medical director who told the surgeon about the 10 percent reward for all costs denied. Managed care of course paints a very different picture from Dr. Peeno's experience and from that depicted in George Anders's book, *Health against Wealth,* which we have referred to frequently. Managed care claims that they only decline to pay for unproven, experimental, or unnecessary procedures and treatments. They say that their purpose is to improve the care of patients by reducing unnecessary or ineffective procedures. They say that, left unsupervised, too many doctors go overboard. They feel that if a cheaper alternative is just as good, using the less expensive one will free resources for other purposes. I believe, as do many of the sources I have studied and as do the great majority of doctors and patients I have interviewed, that the primary purpose of denials is not the altruistic goal they claim, but rather the enhancement of their own profits and their company's stock market valuation. While this may seem a harsh indictment, the plight of the patients whose care they impair is the true condemnation of their practices.

The managed care companies do not tell doctors ahead of time what is acceptable and what is not. The companies use internal sets of guidelines to set their policies, but the actual decisions are up to the doctors and sometimes lesser representatives who field the calls from the doctors requesting approval. There are a number of guidelines, but the most commonly used were developed by a managed care consulting company called Millman and Robertson. They carried out their own analyses of hospital and office records and drew their own conclusions, which are highly controversial. One-day stays for deliveries was one of their recommendations.

When doctors call the HMO for approval of a procedure or treatment, instead of asking what the patient needs, the HMO representative inevitably pushes to find a way for the patient to do without it or to find a cheaper approach. For example, a benefits manager for a small company described to me, on condition of anonymity, some cases he handled. One case involved a young child whose hearing was damaged by an illness in infancy, leaving her little hearing or speech. The pediatrician asked for approval of speech therapy and a hearing aid. The company denied coverage. Their explanation to the doctor was that because the child had never developed speech, due to the early age of the illness, they did not have to provide something the child never had! Another example the benefits manager told me was of a child who had been hit in the face in an accident. She was given various treatments, but the company refused to pay for an ophthalmologist, even though the youngster was hit in the eye and her vision was affected. They said she did not need it, though they never saw or examined her. In still another case, a little girl sustained an injury to her big toe, leaving it disfigured and scarred. The company at first refused to pay for a plastic surgeon because they said, "It just needs to be fixed, it does not matter how it looks."

I am sure that the people making these decisions would give their own children treatment to hear, to speak, to see, and to avoid unsightly scars. Their lust for profits must be considerable if they are willing to make such decisions and statements. When you consult a doctor, you expect to be treated based on the doctor's direct examination of you and on the doctor's skill and experience. Do you really want your doctor's judgement second-guessed by strangers who never see you and whose motives are highly suspect?

An oncologist (cancer specialist) told me recently that he received a call from a managed care nurse questioning the continued hospitalization of one of his patients. He explained that the patient had advanced cancer spread throughout his body, was intubated (a breathing tube down the throat, attached to a respirator), and was in the intensive care unit. There was still some hope of response to the therapy he was getting. The nurse asked many more questions, then finally said that she would approve the stay for another *two* days and then call back. This discussion took a great deal of time away from this very busy doctor. He advised her that nothing was going to change in two days. A patient cannot go from intubation in the ICU to recovery at home in two days! She said she would call back anyway.

There is an endless number of stories of patients who died or suffered grievous complications because of care denied by managed care facilities. I could relate dozens of examples, each worse than the next, but they are included in the references and bibliography for those who wish to review them. As I said in the preface, anecdotes are for illustration only; they are not proof.

Consider instead the issues that lie behind these actions. Dr. Peeno's article and the managed care doctor who told the surgeon of the 10 percent kickback for every denied procedure document what common sense would tell you: *denials are made to save money and increase profit.*

I believe HMOs are in effect practicing medicine, but they say they are only insurance companies deciding payment. Since most people cannot afford medical care without insurance reimbursement, then payment decisions do decide what care the patient gets. I believe that it is unethical to make such important decisions at a distance without examining, speaking to, and knowing the patient.

Remember the description of good medical care: the importance of direct contact, spending time, getting to know patients as whole persons and addressing their unique needs.

"Guidelines" are no way to decide medical need. For example, there is an ongoing concern as to when caesarean deliveries are necessary. Caesarean sections deliver babies surgically when there is reason to believe the baby may be harmed by vaginal delivery. The risk is subject to the obstetrician's judgment, and the use of caesareans varies widely around the country. This variability raised the question whether some or even many may be unnecessary. Yet, to flag all caesareans as suspect and to grill an obstetrician every time one is done makes it harder and harder for the doctor to make a reasoned judgment in each pregnancy.

A second opinion by another, experienced physician can provide a valuable fresh point of view and has been a standard procedure throughout the history of medicine. Second-guessing and micro-managing by a managed care functionary is, in contrast, very hazardous. In the case of managed care, the opinion is not based on careful evaluation of the patient. Instead, it is based on cost considerations and the judgment of people whose first allegiance is to the insurance company, not the patient.

When we walk, we do not think about putting one foot out, then another, then the other, and on and on. If you did, you would walk very clumsily. Think what it would be like if you tried to walk knowing that someone was questioning every step you took. It is the same when others question you excessively, as happens when doctors call managed care companies for approval of tests and treatments.

Let us give managed care the benefit of the doubt that in the beginning the denial process may have at least awakened the profession to look harder at procedures, hospitalizations, and treatments. The idea was to look at everything critically to ensure that the tests and procedures would be effective and necessary, both to spare patients if they weren't and to conserve funds for more effective measures.

That may have been the hope of those whose good intentions have put us on the road to where good intentions often lead, but even if so, there would have been much better ways to do it. To some extent it did awaken doctors to the need to carefully reexamine medical practices to ensure they were worthwhile. By this time, however, the point has been made very effectively and it is no longer necessary to beat patients and doctors over the head with a large sledgehammer.

Very few people are wealthy enough to pay the tens of thousands of dollars required for surgery and hospital costs. For most people, if the insurance does not pay, they cannot afford the test or treatment. In the clinic, I see uninsured people frequently. The clinic charges them a token fee, but any test or procedure done elsewhere is full price and few can find the funds to get the care they need. As I said in a WCBS national news radio interview on April 24, 1998, "The system is not going to work if we say to people, 'We will take care of you when you are healthy or have only minor problems, but don't come to us if you get really sick.' "

Managed care has created a class of people who pay full price for insurance but in reality are underinsured for a significant portion of their needs. They are underinsured because of the cost-shifting we discussed before, the care that is denied, and the impairment of the doctor-patient relationship. If this were being done because we as a nation have limited resources and we have tried to use great wisdom in allocating the funds available, then we would at least have something to consider and develop. However, when decisions are made as a result of greed and desire to gain, hidden from the input of others, there is no benefit to society, only to those few who profit financially at the expense of the many.

The denial process also drains the system in another important way: It is horrendously time consuming and expensive. Doctors usually need extra secretaries just to handle the paperwork and calls involved with seeking approval, justifying treatments, and arguing over denials. Some plans are so understaffed that it can take three or four days for a doctor's office to get past busy signals and endless voice mail to reach a managed care bureaucrat who can hear the problem of one patient, let alone twenty or thirty.[1]

Attempts to reverse a denial require endless additional calls, letters, and more wasted time. Managed care boasts that it reduces administrative burdens. The truth is that it magnifies them many-fold. It is an effective trick—the harder you make it, the more you discourage people from trying. I do no managed care in my private office. I am included on only one managed care panel for the clinic patients (I am paid a salary by the clinic; they do all billing and receive all the funds). Thus, my only direct experience with managed care is for the clinic patients, and that is minimal, but I have learned a great deal about it through research and interviews with physicians and their staffs.

I did get one call about a private patient from his managed care drug plan. It took several tries and considerable time only to find out that they wanted to know if they could substitute a cheaper variant of what I had ordered. It was of no benefit to the patient—in fact, the suggested drug would have been riskier for him—and the sole purpose of the call was to save money for the insurance company. I of course said no, but it cost me considerable wasted time—imagine such a situation magnified hundreds of times, as is true for doctors who participate in managed care.

Doctors who participate in managed care have to belong to many managed care plans, each with its own rules and procedures, each requiring endless forms, reviews, reports, and telephone calls. The administrative burden is enormous, and that does not even include Medicare, which is close to being number one in burdening doctors. Some doctors, such as the Kaiser-Permenente facilities and the HIP (Health Insurance Plan), work for one HMO in the HMO's clinic. They at least have less administrative burden.

Managed care's answer to every effort to dilute their control methods is always that they must keep costs down. Kenneth Abramowitz, a health care analyst for Sanford Bernstein and Co., was asked on CBS (April 24, 1998) about an article noting an increase in HMO premiums. He said, "If society wants to continue to be a bunch of crybabies and demand excess freedom, then insurers will give them that excess freedom and charge them higher rates."[2] He meant that if we force HMOs to liberalize benefits, they will comply but will increase their premiums to cover the increased cost.

Did you know that there could be *excess* freedom? Do you think a mother wanting help for a hearing impaired child is a crybaby? Whom do you want deciding your health care—your doctor or distant Wall Street analysts and executives? Doctors work to make a living and seek profits from their work. The difference is that a doctor deals with you face to face, person to person. Investors do not think of the patients of HMOs as people, they only see the financial figures on paper or computer screens.

Face-to-face, doctors and patients can understand each other, have a feel for each other's needs and beliefs, and work out an approach to the patient's problem that is focused on the unique needs of the patients.

MANAGED CARE'S METHODS MAY CONSTITUTE AN UNETHICAL PRACTICE CALLED FEE SPLITTING

According to the 1997 *Code of Medical Ethics* of the American Medical Association, "Payment by or to a physician for the referral of a patient is fee splitting and unethical."[3] The proscription against fee splitting is universally recognized and adhered to as one of the most important ethical principles in medicine. Recommendations of and by a doctor should be purely on merit without financial interest. Decisions on treatment should be based solely on what is needed for the patient's benefit, not by what is expedient or profitable for the doctor.

In my view, managed care is *de facto* fee splitting. Doctors are given monetary incentives to treat patients in a manner financially beneficial to the insurance company. Doctors are rewarded financially for adhering to those requests. Referrals are based not just on the judgment of the doctor but in compliance with the financial needs of the company. Doctors receive referrals not because of their quality but because they are on a panel arranged by the insurance company. The HMO selects the doctors with whom it contracts to give care. Patients can select their primary doctor only from the HMO doctors, and referrals can be made only from panels of HMO-selected specialists. In some plans the patient can get care outside of the HMO's approved physicians, but at much higher cost.

In a capitation plan, the doctor is in effect rewarded financially for doing less. Care should be based solely on what is right for the patient, not on what is more profitable for the doctor or the insurer.

In a capitation plan, the doctor is paid a fixed amount per patient per year. He receives that amount no matter what he does, so the less he does for the patient, the more money he retains. Managed care companies claim this is an incentive to keep patients healthy, but it obviously is equally an incentive to do as little as possible.

An insurance company should be only an agent for managing money. Insurance companies should not be in the business of deciding care based on their own profit needs. By involving themselves in decisions about care of the patient in a way that redounds to their financial benefit, they are splitting the fee with the doctor.

I believe managed care is an unethical form of fee splitting. I am not aware of any statements by the AMA, the American College of Physicians, or any other agency that establishes standards of ethics on this subject. I believe they should consider it.

The managed care companies and their supporters would argue they do not reward doctors who do less, but simply encourage efficient care. I believe that there is overwhelming evidence of the hypocrisy of this view. It is as if a policeman holds a gun to the suspect's head to make him confess, then later says that he simply asked the prisoner to tell the truth.

The medical associations that formulate ethics guidelines have not spoken on this issue. I believe the medical establishment has felt the inevitability of the fiscal power of corporations and in frustration has tried to make the best of things. It is similar to the situation with tobacco. Banning tobacco is so politically dangerous that no one wants to touch the issue. Tobacco use and products have been specifically exempted from the jurisdiction of the FDA and the Consumer Products Safety Commission (CPSC).

If the FDA were to rule on tobacco, the greatest cause of death and disease in this country and soon to be for the whole world, by the same criteria as it does any other drug, the FDA would either ban it completely or at least apply the same kinds of restrictions it applies to heroin and cocaine. If the CPSC ruled on tobacco, it would ban it as a product that is extremely dangerous when used as it is designed to be used and which cannot be made safe.

The two industries, managed care and tobacco, have much in common. They are both highly profit-driven at the expense of consumers, they both wield enormous power by virtue of their size and wealth, they both expend huge sums in lobbying congress for protection, and they both engender sizable hostile opposition among major segments of the population.

It is thus not surprising that the major medical associations are in a bind as to how to deal with such a powerful force that now controls so much of the income of their members.

The American Medical Association was badly hurt by their opposition to universal Medicare coverage (they advocated coverage for the *needy* elderly), a stand which we now see was the absolutely correct position, since Medicare is going broke trying to cover everyone. Nevertheless, they are beginning to speak out increasingly forcefully against managed care, concerned as they are that they will be wrongly accused of simply trying to preserve doctors' welfare. Some physician organizations have attempted to determine how best to live with managed care. I do not think we should try to accommodate managed care, because I do not think we can compromise with ethics.

I suspect that large organizations suffer from *committee-itis*. People behave differently in committees and in institutional politics. Being on a committee changes how people think. The field of study of group dynamics, how people behave in groups, has amply described how beliefs and decisions are strongly affected by group pressures and interactions. As an example of committee-itis, I remember consulting for a large corporation about a conflict between an older clerk and a young supervisor. The supervisor wanted to move the clerk out of a supply storeroom and into a messenger job around the office. The older woman refused and the young supervisor wanted her fired. I examined the clerk at some length and the story became apparent. She was a Holocaust survivor and was suffering from Holocaust Survivor Syndrome. While all survivors carry scars and seldom stop having nightmares, some can never recover enough from the unspeakable horrors to which they were exposed. This woman found it very difficult to deal with people, but for decades had happily found a niche in her safe little storeroom. The twenty-five-year-old supervisor did not need to move the sixty-three-year-old clerk, but when I spoke with the supervisor, it was obvious that she viewed it as a power struggle and a challenge to her new authority. I then advised the personnel officer of my findings. He understood, felt compassion for the human elements involved, and promised to work with the supervisor to resolve things so the woman could remain where she had been for so long.

I saw him the following week. His whole manner had changed. With an officious voice he told me that he had presented it to the committee that decides such things and that for the sake of order and authority the Holocaust survivor was being fired. He would no longer listen to discussion. His eyes had the blank look of a man who has retreated into the protective arms of a committee. He needed the security of a group decision just as the Holocaust survivor needed the security of a known situation, but I think one of them had a much more deserving need.

The Holocaust survivor was fired. She had somehow survived the concentration camp, but her job could not survive a committee. A word of warning: Beware of committees. They have no heart and soul. They may sometimes be correct, but are they right?

Science and medicine do not work well by committee or by organizational politics. The search for truth cannot be conducted by committee vote. The whole purpose of science is, to the best degree possible, to divorce truth-finding from opinion, belief, desire, convenience, or anything else that detracts from completely objective observation.

Some medical organizations are contributing valuable work

toward the issues we are discussing. I feel, however—and I think I represent a very large percentage of practicing physicians—that many have not been strong enough in their opposition to managed care's intrusion on medical practice. I strongly suspect that many officials of these organizations, if they were free to react individually, would be closer to the point of view I have outlined.

MANAGED CARE FINDS WAYS TO INSURE ONLY HEALTHY PEOPLE, THOUGH THEY PRESENT THEMSELVES AS UNIVERSAL INSURERS FOR EVERYONE

It is easy to insure healthy young people cheaply. It is the same reason stores love to sell service contracts on modern audio equipment, which rarely breaks down. Managed care is marketed to those with the least need for expensive care. It is what sold corporations on them in the first place—seemingly inexpensive insurance. The insurance companies would weed out those with higher utilization rates by cancelling contracts or denying so much care that sicker patients had to look elsewhere. The companies did not mind because there were plenty of young healthy bodies left to replace them. But as managed care's share of the market increased the profitability of managed care is declining. They have so penetrated the market that they have exhausted the supply of young, healthy customers and they can no longer afford to have a high turnover rate among subscribers, since the competition for members has become fierce.

Notice also that the insurance companies are beginning to backpedal on the rush to take over Medicare and Medicaid patients. Those pesky old people and those poor folk have the nerve to actually get sick! Managed care does not like sick people. They require more care and are more expensive to have in the system.

There have been discussions about "futile" care recently. If you read between the lines, what they are really saying is why can't these people just die quickly and save us money? Someone came up with one of those very convenient statistics that more money is spent on the last six months of life than on the whole of life prior to that period. I doubt if that applies to very many people. Use your own common sense. Do you really think more is spent in six months than in most people's *whole* life? Even if someone spends a few weeks in an ICU and builds up a huge bill, that doesn't mean that we should not try to save our loved ones. Certainly there is a point at which prolonging life artificially only prolongs suffering. Where we draw the line is a deeply personal decision that should be based on humanity, not cost.

Recently a friend faced exactly such a situation and called me about it several times. His father was in an apparent coma with a severe, disfiguring infection, in an apparently hopeless condition. Even if his father recovered, his abilities would be severely limited. The son grieved for him and felt his father would not want to live that way, but his mother could not bring herself to make the decision to take her husband off life-support. Eventually, time resolved it for both.

Should the mother have been forced to tell doctors to end her husband's life? We know that stopping support in a hopeless condition is different than ending a life, but when it is *your* hand on the respirator switch, it doesn't always feel merciful.

I took care of a sixty-year-old man who, on his first visit to me, was experiencing a leg pain that was very difficult to diagnose—until we finally found the cancer in his pelvis that was pressing on a nerve and causing the pain. (We never found the cause, which can happen with this type of cancer, but it did not matter because it was already too far advanced to make a difference.) He was a highly intelligent, warm man with a close and loving family. They wanted time together before what they knew would be the ultimate outcome, so we began intensive treatment. It was hard on him and there were the usual complications and side effects. At one point he seemed to slip into a coma and was intubated and on various forms of life support in the ICU. Looking at this man, anyone would have said it was hopeless, let him go, do not waste money, and all the rest.

I felt differently. I had eight specialists on his case and saw the patient several times a day, coordinating everything. Each specialist did his or her job, but coordination was essential, as always. If no one is taking care of the patient, only taking care of his organs, disaster results. Every day I spoke to him, comforted him, and explained all that was happening to him, although he never responded and he looked terrible. Even his family felt he was too deeply unconscious to be aware of their presence.

Then one day he began to improve and we were able to take him off the life support. He was fully awake. He later told me that he had heard and understood everything I had told him. Though no one else had talked to him, my conversation was enough to keep him going, to keep him sane throughout the long ordeal.

He went home to his family and lived another six months, time which his family said meant a lot to him and to them.

How do we put a price on a life? How do we decide for another person when to say goodbye? We can gently counsel, we can listen and we can comfort, but we must not play God. We will discuss in chapter 10 how best to allocate our limited resources, but such decisions must never be made by those whose only interest is profit. If it is your father in that bed, you want help from those who care, not those who only count money.

WASTE AND FRAUD ARE CONTROLLED TOO TIGHTLY

President George Bush was jogging one day and collapsed. He was found to have an irregular heart rhythm called atrial fibrillation (AF). AF is due to several possible causes, one of which is an overactive thyroid gland. The thyroid sits at the base of your neck below the Adam's apple and releases hormones that regulate your body's metabolic rate, as well as affecting many other important functions.

Thyroid dysfunction is easily detectable by simple, inexpensive blood tests and the president is the most medically watched and examined man in America. Yet, here was the leader of the free world nearly killed by a condition that could have been detected much earlier by a simple blood test. How did this happen? According to the newspapers, his doctors were saving money by not doing a wasteful test.

Much testing is being challenged by a new technique called a cost-effectiveness study. You do a test on a group of people, find the ones who have the disease the test screens for and then see for how many testing actually made a difference (i.e., affected the outcome of the disease through early diagnosis). You then divide the cost of testing the whole group by the number of people who benefitted, and the result per person tells you the cost of achieving that benefit.

Then there is cost-benefit analysis, which can be used to ask: Is it cheaper to perform a test or procedure or not to perform it? That is, will testing everyone prevent enough expense of illness in the minority whose results show that they have the disease to justify paying for doing the test on everyone? Suppose a company spends $100,000 to screen a large group of people for disease X. It finds ten people with the disease. Undetected until much later, their care would have cost the company $80,000. It costs only $20,000 to treat them all at the early stage detected by the screening test.

The company would then spend $100,000 on screening plus $20,000 on early treatment, for a total expenditure of $120,000. If the screening program is not implemented, the only expense would be

$80,000 for treating those not found until late in their disease. That means that it would cost the company $40,000 more to detect the disease at an early state. The ten people would benefit greatly by the early detection. The company would have to decide if it wanted to spend an extra $40,000 to help those ten people at an earlier stage of the disease.

Large corporations have been accused of making just such calculations in other ways. For example, if a company discovers a defect in its product that will result in death to a small number of customers, their economists can calculate for them the cost of the resulting lawsuits versus the cost of correcting the defect. The accusations have been made that the companies leave the defect uncorrected because settling the suits would be cheaper. That would mean they deliberately allowed people to die because it was cheaper than preventing those deaths.

That is an incredibly serious indictment if true. Since I have no direct knowledge of the accuracy of these charges, I will not identify the accused companies. However, that the choice even exists means that there will be those companies that will at least be tempted. Now suppose the adverse outcome is very bad but not quite as clear-cut as, say, a death in an accident from a correctable defect. Then one can easily begin to rationalize, to tell oneself that it really is not important and to pursue the cheap way.

Returning to President Bush's case, apparently the learned experts issued guidelines for screening tests that did not include thyroid tests. The president's doctors, being in the government, reportedly did not include them in the panel of tests on the president, even though his health is considered by most of us to be critical to our country—and his own wife has been treated for the same disease! Fortunately, Bush survived and should do perfectly well, but it was a close call that could have come out much worse. I never blindly trust reports in newspapers and I hope that there is a more plausible explanation for how this occurred. Perhaps Bush actually had the test at an earlier time when his thyroid was still normal.

Even if this story is apocryphal, the process is not, however. This very kind of cost calculation and planning is affecting the care that *you* receive from your doctor. While it is vital to use our resources wisely, how to do so is much more complicated than a simple cost-effectiveness calculation. Cost effectiveness is a limited tool that must be used with great caution and must never replace individual judgment. Unfortunately, I believe profiteers and planners have jumped at the chance to use such a tool that can be easily manipulated and cited to support their point of view.

One can be fairly certain that if it is cheaper not to do a test than to do it, managed care will choose not to perform the test. That would be all right *if* price were all that mattered. And it would seem that for the companies, price *is* all that matters. For you and me, however, there is much more at stake.

The most important point right now is "What counts as waste?" One person's waste is another's necessity. Recall that an early admission to the hospital was termed a "creature comfort" for the eighty-year-old man in Linda Peeno's article. Another example would be air-conditioning. Is it a creature comfort? For a healthy twenty-year-old it is. For a frail seventy-year-old it is a necessity, as it is for a severe asthmatic or a premature baby just home from the hospital. For these patients, a hot, humid environment can be anywhere from debilitating to fatal.

I was recently asked to assist in the appeal for a very ill clinic patient to remain at home with home attendants rather than be forced into a nursing home. He is an eighty-seven-year-old Hasidic rabbi who has many diseases and disabilities, but he functions at a reasonable level in his home, where he has lived for many decades. The home attendant knows his needs and preferences, how to get him to eat and be more active, and other small but vital aspects of his lifestyle. The rabbi has no family left but friends and neighbors visit him and one has taken on the job of being his advocate.

Despite previous scandals and revelations about nursing homes, governmental and newspaper studies have revealed continued shockingly poor conditions and care at as many as 61 percent of nursing homes. While some are excellent, in the poor-quality facilities the staffs are often limited and poorly trained and supervised. They have little time for patient care. Patients are frequently neglected and treated heartlessly.[4] Under such conditions the rabbi would quickly deteriorate to a vegetative state. Is it a "waste" of taxpayers' money to keep him in the home he has known for decades, cared for by an aide and the community?

Consider the heart patient sent home after three days only to suffer a heart attack and have to be rushed back, much worse off. The extra days in the hospital that managed care felt were wasteful would have *saved* money—and *her* health.

Cutting truly wasteful tests and procedures is by definition a goal of which we all approve. However, if the cutting of waste is not done carefully with concern for patients, you really can throw out the baby with the bath water. Redundancy and a little waste are sometimes needed to avoid error. Cutting too close to the edge is courting disaster.

Suppose you own an airplane. You bear the entire cost of running your plane and you have a limited budget. You are advised to spend extra money to install several backup systems on your plane and a grizzled old-timer says, "Sonny, always have extra gas in your tanks."

Airplane fuel is very expensive and all those gadgets cost a fortune. You decide you know best and refuse all the extras because you do not want to waste money. Now you are flying happily up above trees and then things begin to go wrong. Instruments fail but you have no backup. You wander off course and run out of gas. You crash-land and survive by the skin of your teeth, but the damage to your plane and to structures on the ground costs you 100 times more than the backup systems and extra gas would have.

In medicine, the risks are great. Paring down to the bone is penny-wise and pound-foolish. Depth, leeway, backup, and redundancy of diagnostic procedures, treatment options, and monitoring methods are essential to good care.

Medicare is following the same pattern now as managed care, increasingly restricting procedures and tests that Medicare unilaterally decides are wasteful.

Medicare now requires a diagnosis code to accompany every test ordered or it will not pay for the test. If Medicare disagrees with the doctor's choice of code, it can charge the doctor with *fraud* and assess very high penalties. The book of codes is hundreds of pages of very small type. The codes can often have dozens of subheadings. There are three digits, a decimal point and two more digits; each digit subcategorizes the condition. For example, hepatitis: which kind, acute or chronic, active or inactive, major or minor, and on and on.

Then there are the procedure codes, which are equally involved, but in a different way. There are fewer procedure codes, but much more stringent requirements as to what is written in the chart to justify them. The codes for office visits specify how much time in minutes, what organs should be covered, how serious are the problems, and the like.

Will there be an army of inspectors invading doctors' offices routing out the evil miscoders? Medicare and the president have launched major campaigns to eliminate waste and fraud. Much of the fraud they are referring to relates to disputes over coding diagnoses and procedures. This is not fraud. Some doctors bill for work they never did—*that* is fraud. But the massive estimates of the cost of fraud include coding errors and differences of opinion.

The news media report cases of fraud very prominently. Though they represent a tiny fraction of the medical profession, the public hears only about those few who cheat, and it sullies their perception of all doctors. (One could argue that the abuses of a few HMOs or of some of their employees do not invalidate the whole system. I agree, but in the case of managed care the abuses are widespread and the system itself is inherently flawed.) This situation also raises an important question: Should we create an ever more burdensome bureaucracy that results in diminishing marginal returns just to catch the small minority who abuse the system? Should we diminish the quality of care for all to punish the few?

What are all these codes for? Is a liver function test valid if the disease is acute but not if it is chronic? Will the experts in Washington decide how often Mrs. Jones in Tuscaloosa should have a liver test? Every eight weeks is okay but every seven weeks is fraud? Each bureaucrat says he or she just needs this code or that additional detail and it will only take a moment for the doctor to comply. All those little moments add up to a crushing burden.

Coding has become a major industry with very expensive books, seminars, and newsletters designed to help doctors code correctly. Some of the instruction teaches doctors how to code to maximize their reimbursement. It is like a chess match between Medicare and doctors, full of strategy and subterfuge on both sides.

Medicare sets the pattern for all other insurers. If doctors were to comply fully with all the requirements, they would spend more time on coding, note writing, reports, referrals, and other paperwork for their multitude of masters than they would on patient care. (If we could just get those patients out of the picture, then we would have time to do the paperwork!) The managed care story is especially disturbing because most of the cost savings are not for society's benefit or yours, but for the benefit of the managed care company!

MANAGED CARE HAS DEMORALIZED PHYSICIANS AND REDUCED THEM FROM INDEPENDENT PROFESSIONALS TO THE EQUIVALENT OF EMPLOYEES TIGHTLY CONTROLLED BY THEIR EMPLOYERS

Why do bright, high achieving students go into medicine? They could do much better in business, law, or finance with no physical risk. (Medicine is much riskier than most people realize: exposure to life-threatening, contagious infectious diseases; risks of HIV, hepatitis, and other diseases from needle sticks; psychotic patients; long hours of physically and emotionally exhausting work; high stress; and easy accessibility to drugs.) In all the surveys I have read, the main appeal of medicine as a career is the opportunity to help people. These students express the need to have an important purpose in their lives.

The second most important reason seems to be independence. After that comes the intellectual challenge, the glamour of surgery, prestige, the job security, the flexibility, and the income. The last varies in importance but most people want to earn a good living and medicine used to provide that.

Modern medical students seem prepared for the different world into which they will graduate. They *think* they are prepared. They do not realize how bad things really are. Almost every doctor I have spoken to would advise prospective doctors *against* entering medicine today.

Published surveys seldom reflect the depth of unhappiness among physicians. Yet the American College of Physicians (ACP) recently published a preliminary report of a new survey it will be publishing (full results not available as of this writing) in which "about 90 percent of internists surveyed by telephone last fall reported that they were satisfied with their careers."[5] Those who liked managed care cited autonomy, quality of health care and reduced paperwork; those who did not, cited *loss* of autonomy, heavy bureaucracy, and limits on referrals.

These results are very different from what I have heard in all my interviews and found in my review of the literature. In a personal communication, I have been advised by one of the ACP executives that nearly all of the doctors reached by the survey were those who had profitable managed care practices! Obviously, it is a skewed sample.

A far more realistic study was recently published. It reported a survey of over 1,000 Pennsylvania primary care physicians. The study found that "Many physicians surveyed believe managed care has significant negative effects on the physician-patient relationship, the ability to carry out ethical obligations, and on quality of patient care."[6]

Let us consider the assaults on a physician's psyche:

1. *Loss of autonomy:* physicians used to be the sole arbiters of all health care for the sole benefit of their patients. Now their power is usurped by clerks, bureaucrats, lawyers, administrators, laws, guidelines, competitive "providers," and managed care agents. Cost is the only criterion that seems to matter. While most doctors were once solo practitioners by choice, they have been forced into group practices as the only way to survive in the managed care world. While groups have

some advantages, for many it means the loss of the independence and freedom of solo practice. Economists, planners, quality controllers, and endless streams of experts of all kinds have created a new industry, the second-guess-the-doctor industry, to study everything they do.

Doctors by nature are highly independent—it is one of the things that puts the science in medicine. Truth is not found by consensus, it is found by objective observation of the experienced world. Doctors are terrible team players. They feel very passionately, are of necessity obsessive and compulsive about their work (outside of work they can be as much a slob as the next person), and are totally unimpressed by authorities whose views are not supported by objective evidence. The new managed care medicine is stealing the cherished independence of medicine. We should note in this discussion of loss of doctors' autonomy that patients are also losing their autonomy as managed care intrudes on their lives and controls the care they receive. Your choices in your own health care decisions are more limited under managed care than ever in the past.

2. *Intimidation:* Deviance from the "experts' " mandated procedures entails the threat of what may be unfounded malpractice suits, penalties, and fines in legal actions; prosecution for fraud; and expulsion from participation under Medicare, Medicaid, and contracts under managed care. Surveillance of doctors has escalated to unprecedented proportions. A national data bank of transgressors has been set up and every year hours are spent filling out credentialing forms repeatedly asking the same information.

In 1985, Congress passed the Consolidated Omnibus Budget Reconciliation Act (COBRA), which included health care provisions among many others. Included was a provision engineered by Rep. Fortney H. Stark (D-Calif.) that prohibited doctors from referring patients to facilities in which they had a financial interest. Two years later, Medicare sent a survey asking doctors to report any such financial interest. The deadline for returning the survey was one month.

The fine for submitting it late was *$10,000 per day* for *each day* past the one-month deadline! No one believes this when I tell them, but here is an exact quote from Empire Blue Cross Blue Shield (the Medicare administrator in New York) in its Medicare Bulletin 91–16, July 1991: "Section 1877(g) of the Social Security Act prescribes a civil money penalty of up to $10,000 for each day after October 1, 1991, that the required survey information is delayed."

They had waited two years to send the survey, so it obviously was not urgent. What other reason could there be for such an absurdly severe penalty than to impress doctors with the power the government wields over them?

There is another law, usually applied to multibillion-dollar defense contractors, that can be applied to doctors who simply choose a different code than the government thinks appropriate. It is called the False Claims Act and dates from the Civil War.[7] As applied to doctors a false claim is any bill for services submitted to Medicare that is found to be incorrect. Today it carries a $5,000 to $10,000 penalty per each false claim plus triple damages and costs. There need be no *intent* to defraud, only that the contractor *should* have known that the claim (billing) would be considered false. Even if the billing was a simple mistake, under law it can be considered fraudulent. All bills submitted to insurers, including Medicare, must today have a code number that designates the diagnosis that justifies the service for which the doctor is charging a fee.

Thus derives the "fraud" terminology for alleged coding violations. If a doctor thinks a patient *might* have diabetes and tests for that, the government could, at least by the letter of the law, prosecute the doctor for fraud for ordering a test for a disease the doctor did not yet know the patient had. The government has recently set certain criteria for "correctly" billing by specifying which diagnostic codes justify tests or what kind of service justifies a procedure. As you can imagine, a doctor may reasonably interpret need differently from the government, since obviously experts can disagree with each other on many issues. In 1987 one doctor was convicted under this law for submitting thirty-nine false claims totaling $549.04. He had to pay $79,098.08. The penalties were lower then—today his total penalty would be a staggering $586,647.12![8]

Medicare sets the fees for doctors and some states limit the fees further. The doctor may not charge one penny above the allowed fee. The penalty for any "overcharge" above one dollar is up to a *$2,000* fine and expulsion from Medicare. That is for *each* claim that violates the limit. Fortunately, so far the government seems to reserve this for high volumes of overcharges. These penalties arose in response to fraud committed by a very small number of doctors in the past. The system created to catch the few is penalizing the many, both doctors and their patients, by distorting the practice of Medicine.

How often have these penalties been imposed? There were over three thousand prosecutions in 1997.[9] Considering the number of doctors and the huge volume of claims, that is a small number, but probably still more than necessary. More important than the numbers is that the *threat* of them exists. They exert a chilling effect on the open practice of medicine. The heavy hand of government has ruined many lives in many other areas, even those who are eventually found innocent. Fear of prosecution can distort medical care just as much as fear of being sued for malpractice.

I believe that the vast majority of doctors are honest, and honest doctors despise the small minority who cheat. True fraud should be found and punished, but do we really want to put our entire force of healers under excessive scrutiny and threat just to weed out a small minority of abusers? I believe that the estimates of fraud are badly exaggerated and that this is as much an attempt to constrain costs by any means as it is a valid attempt to limit fraud. Unfortunately, there is no way to prove who is right, and Medicare wields the power of the government. This is another reason why I recommend an entirely new system of health care in the last chapter. If medical associations were given the opportunity to take over fraud control from the government, they would do it very well to avoid the government needing to come back in.

The end does *not* justify the means. That seems to be a lesson we must relearn every day.

3. *Loss of patient loyalty and contact:* One of the joys of medicine is developing long-standing relationships with patients. As you grow and age with your patients, as you share their joys and tragedies, as you see the benefits you bring them, as you see their lives unfold over many years, there is a satisfaction and reward to be found here that exists in few other endeavors. But today, patient populations turn over constantly because so many employers keep changing the plans they make available to their employees. If your current doctor does not participate in the new plan, as is often the case, you have to find a new doctor. In addition, time with patients has shrunk to a shadow of what it once was. Doctors and patients seldom have time any more to get to know each other and build trust and cooperation.

The doctor-patient relationship has gone from one of trust to one that is adversarial as patients blame the doctor for the loss of their benefits. The managed care plans promise their clients everything; their ads paint a rosy picture and the brochures list all kinds of benefits. The plans do not tell the patient that they do not provide the means to deliver what they promise. For example, as we noted previously, they depict a primary care doctor who gives you most of your care and coordinates the rest, but they do not pay the primary care doctors enough to allow adequate time to do all that.

They leave it to the doctor to reveal the reality to the patient, to expose the empty promises. Some managed care companies have gag clauses that prevent the doctor from criticizing the company or even advising the patient of available options outside of the plan.

Each state has its own rules that allow or limit gag clauses. New York is more limiting. An example of a gag clause in a contract for a New York State HMO reads as follows:

> Primary Care Physician agrees that all written material describing [the HMO]'s quality improvement, risk management and utilization management programs, including, but not limited to: *The Provider Guide*; peer review programs; credentialing procedures; complaint procedures; and any other protocols and procedures developed by or for [the HMO] is proprietary information that shall not be disclosed to anyone who is not employed by [the HMO] or directly involved in the performance of this agreement.

Many companies understandably seek to keep information on their internal procedures private to prevent competitors from using them or capitalizing on them in some other way. However, in this case, it means that their subscribers are prevented from knowing how important decisions about their care are made, procedures that might affect their privacy, contractual arrangements the doctor is under that may affect his or her decisions, and other such factors that they should be entitled to know.

In the past, and most likely still existing in some states, were gag clauses that prohibited the doctor from even telling the patient about treatments and resources that had not been approved by the HMO. That meant that if the doctor knew of a better treatment but the HMO did not allow it, the doctor was not supposed to tell the patient about it. The patient might want to seek alternative ways to get that treatment, but would have no way of knowing to look for them.

The patients cannot yell at a faceless corporation so they vent their anger at the doctors and other medical staff. Patients today see the doctor as the barrier they must surmount to get the care they feel they need and deserve.

4. *A doctor may be as much as $150,000 in debt from student loans by the time of graduation.* To be a specialist requires four years of college with very high marks to get into medical school, four years of medical school, a year of hospital duty and a huge exam to be licensed, two to seven years of postgraduate hospital training, and more massive exams to be recognized as a specialist. Specialties include the "primary care"

fields of internal medicine, family practice, pediatrics, and obstetrics-gynecology, as well as surgery, medical subspecialties, and many others. I believe I can speak for every doctor: We did not go through all the years of training, all the hard work that follows, the long hours, the exhaustion, the risks, the stress, the lost nights, the lost time with our families—all that just to make profits for businesspeople who have inserted themselves between us and our patients!

I believe that police officers and firefighters are among the underpaid and underappreciated members of society. They risk their lives for us and work under terrible conditions. They are among the most important members of the community. I believe they should be paid and respected far better than they are. However, those who want to join either force know before they sign up that they are joining an organization and that they will have to comply, military-fashion, with the rules and the pay scale. They know that there can be no independent practitioners.

Physicians, however, enter their field with the full understanding that they do not have to belong to anything and that they are free to practice any way they wish as long as they meet ethical and proficiency standards. I can't think of another profession in which the government changed the rules in the middle of the game. As we discussed previously, doctors have in effect been forced into employment as much as if they were on a direct government payroll.

Medicine is now the only segment of the economy on which wage and price controls are imposed. During the Nixon administration the president enforced such controls on the entire country in an ill-fated experiment in the 1970s to reduce inflation. The wage and price controls slowed inflation temporarily but distorted the economy so badly that they were soon abandoned. I remember vividly the unhappiness with the controls felt by all segments of the population. Even if wage and price controls seem like the easy solution, they create more problems than they solve. Imagine how it feels to be the *only* Americans so treated today.

Most doctors live up to their professional standards and they tend to be fairly positive in attitude generally (you pretty much have to be to survive dealing with disease and injury every day). Can this last under such duress? Experience is invaluable in medicine. We get better every day and with every patient. The study of medicine never ends. There are always new challenges. One of the major casualties of the new economics is that senior doctors, the ones most experienced, the ones with the greatest accumulated wisdom, are leaving medicine. This phenomenon has become a major brain drain. I know firsthand from my many interviews that doctors are very unhappy with today's health care system. This dissatisfaction can be missed or misrepresented by incorrectly structured surveys of physicians.

Surveys like the ACP survey above in which they questioned many physicians who did well financially in managed care can be misleading by their skewed selection of respondents and by the way the questions are asked.

A lot depends on how questions are phrased. Suppose you ask, "All things considered, are you happy with your choice of a career?" If a doctor looks back over his or her whole career, most doctors will remember the satisfactions and rewards, especially since most had a number of years before managed care. But if you ask if the doctor is satisfied with all the changes in managed care, then the answer would likely be very different. Examine the studies carefully and do not trust media simplifications, just as you know to be skeptical about advertising and political claims. A good pollster can finesse the question to come up with any answer desired.

This is important because managed care and its proponents cite endless surveys about patient satisfaction and doctor satisfaction. *Newsweek* published an excellent article analyzing the quality of these surveys and exposing the many flaws in their methodology.[10]

Author Ellyn Spragins points out first of all that most of the surveys managed care companies feature in their ads are satisfaction surveys—how many subscribers to their health insurance plans are satisfied with the plan. She notes that satisfaction does not guarantee quality. Most people are in no position to measure the quality of the care that the company is providing them. They may like the building and the drug plan, but that does not mean they are getting good care.

Secondly, she reports that the surveys are conducted almost entirely among healthy people. Someone who visits a doctor a few times a year for minor problems has little to complain about. When people who have chronic diseases or who have had serious diseases or injuries are surveyed separately, studies have shown that the satisfaction rates plummet. The measure of a health plan is how it takes care of you when you have a serious condition, not when it handles the easy, minor problems.

Even the satisfaction rating itself is misleading, for the companies arrive at their high ratings by lumping together those who are very satisfied, somewhat satisfied and just satisfied and thus can make claims like Tufts Health Plan's "99% member satisfaction." The ads feature similar kinds of claims for many of the companies.

Decide for yourself whether you think doctors are happy about the current medical system. Decide for yourself whether patients are happy—that is, the ones who actually need care, not those whose only exposure has been for a cold or a minor injury.

If you are one who has been well and has not needed much, remember that that could change at any moment. The purpose of insurance is to be there when you need it. You hope you will never need it, but you pay a great deal of money to be prepared. Do you feel you will receive all that you need if the time comes?

NOTES

1. George Anders, *Health against Wealth, HMOs and the Breakdown of Medical Trust* (New York: Houghton Mifflin, 1996).
2. WCBS National news, April 24, 1998.
3. American Medical Association, *Code of Medical Ethics, 1996–1997 Edition* (Chicago: AMA, 1997).
4. Frederick U. Dicker and Greg Birnbaum, "Hellish Abuse at City Nursing Homes," *New York Post* (March 15, 1997): 8–9; Mark Thompson, "Shining a Light on Abuse," *Time* 152 (August 3, 1998): 42–44.
5. American College of Physicians, "Despite Managed Care, Internists Are Satisfied," *ACP Observer* 18 (March 1998): 1.
6. Debra S. Feldman, Dennis H. Novack, and Edward Gracely, "Effects of Managed Care on Physician-Patient Relationships, Quality of Care, and the Ethical Practice of Medicine," *Archives of Internal Medicine* 158 (August 10 and 24, 1998): 1626–32.
7. William S. Fein, "The Federal False Claims Act," *Unique Opportunities* (May/June 1995): 9–12.
8. Ibid.
9. "Newswatch," *Internal Medicine World Report* 13 (January 15–31, 1998): 1.
10. Ellen E. Spragins, "The Numbers Racket," *Newsweek* (May 5, 1997): 77.

8

Privacy

The right of the people to be secure in their persons, houses, papers, and effects, against unreasonable searches and seizures, shall not be violated, and no warrants shall issue, but upon probable cause, supported by oath or affirmation, and particularly describing the place to be searched, and the persons or things to be seized.

—The Fourth Amendment to the
Constitution of the United States

As we discussed in chapter 2, privacy is essential to the doctor-patient relationship. Because personal information is crucial to good care, patients must feel confident that they can discuss even their most embarrassing history, intimate secrets, and feelings without fear of disclosure.

Privacy is a critical issue in all of medicine and our concern in this book is not just managed care but, equally important, what would be the best health care system we could devise. Any system we adopt must protect privacy fully and consistently. The problems we are about to discuss are not unique to managed care, but they are exacerbated by managed care methods. Managed care regularly inserts itself into the doctor-patient relationship more than any other entity, other than perhaps a criminal investigation, and managed care uses new, intensive methods to monitor medical practice.

There are many legitimate reasons for access to medical records. Regulatory agencies designed to protect patients by detecting substandard medical practice need access to the record to investigate suspected doctors. Law enforcement agents need access when investigating possible crimes. All the people involved in your care, such as other doctors, nurses, various therapists, and so on, need to look at your chart.

Since fraud and abuse to obtain insurance benefits falsely have been present since insurance began, the medical record is the primary evidence used to help control this illegal activity. Not only are fraud and abuse illegal and unethical, in practical terms they affect us all because they significantly increase the cost of insurance for everyone. Insurers need some way to verify that claims are legitimate and appropriate for reimbursement. Every health insurance policy requires that the insured must sign an agreement to release medical information.

Much valuable medical research can be conducted by reviewing charts. Pharmaceutical companies use chart review in evaluating the safety and effectiveness of drugs. Epidemiologists look for patterns that suggest new diseases or environmental or other causes for diseases. Scientists in many fields use records to study large numbers of people in pursuit of their area of research. Infectious disease experts look for information to combat contagious diseases. Health economists look for ways to improve health care delivery. Employers use medical records to guide their benefits programs and to reassure themselves that their benefit dollars are being used properly.

Marketing companies eagerly seek all kinds of medical information to target sales efforts. Pharmaceutical companies, which have taken over many medication distribution companies, use prescription records to target sales pitches for their products. For example, if you take a cholesterol-lowering drug, you might receive a mailing or telemarketing call urging you to ask your doctor to switch to the seller's brand. Two huge pharmacy chains admitted to sharing their computer records of your prescriptions with pharmaceutical marketing companies. The companies quickly "suspended" (does that mean they might later be reinstated?) this practice when exposed in the news media, but seek other ways to target potential customers.

Insurance company drug plans for some time now have required doctors to give the pharmacy their DEA number for *every* prescription whether a restricted drug or not. The DEA is the federal Drug Enforcement Agency, which controls the prescription and use of what are called "controlled substances," which are mainly tranquilizers, narcotics, and similar drugs that have a high addiction potential. Each doctor is assigned a number required for every controlled substance prescription. The DEA instructs doctors to reveal their DEA number *only* when prescribing controlled substances, but most patients will not be able to get a drug through their HMO drug plan, since they require the DEA number be attached to every prescription. The HMOs and pharmaceutical companies use the DEA number as a universal physician identifier which allows them to track every prescription every doctor writes and to monitor what prescriptions are being filled by every pharmacy.

I inquired once of the DEA as to how we physicians were to resolve their instructions to restrict use of the number and the patients' need to get their prescriptions filled. The agent told me that they were well aware of the problem but had no plans either to resolve it or to change their instructions for physicians. A corollary to this is that in New York State all controlled substance prescriptions are reported to the state's control agency. The worthwhile purpose of this is to control sale of prescriptions to drug abusers and drug dealers. The downside is that if you are taking a tranquilizer or some other controlled drug prescribed for you legally by your doctor, that information is in yet another computer.

Managed care has additional reasons to obtain information. Their stated goal is to improve the management of their clients' medical care, to spare those clients unnecessary or harmful practices and procedures, to ensure sensible utilization of medical resources, to gather data, information and experience to improve their own methods, and to ensure as well that their money is being used wisely and frugally. They must be able to access the medical records and to question doctors in detail to accomplish these goals. Since they take upon themselves the stated responsibility to "manage" their clients' care, which is what the term "managed care" is intended to mean, they have escalated the degree of gathering information about patients far beyond what was ever done by insurance companies in the past.

Under the old, traditional indemnity plans (the ones that simply reimburse bills), the primary check on appropriateness was the diagnosis that the doctor would write on the bill or requisition for a procedure. Occasionally, payment of bills was denied with a letter requesting more information, which, when supplied by the doctor in a brief note, usually resulted in approval. Toward the end of these plans' heyday, as costs were rising steeply, denials and letters were used increasingly, but indemnity plans never resorted to the much more intrusive methods employed by managed care.

HMOs have created the practice of using patient records to track which patients are receiving preventive measures, such as mammograms and PAP smears, to improve compliance. They use these lists to notify doctors to contact patients who are not up-to-date and to send doctors information on these practices. While that is an admirable goal, nevertheless it constitutes a further encroachment on patients' autonomy.

HMOs instituted a whole new scale of involvement in patient information. They use increasingly sophisticated computer programs to track and collect data. They employ an army of doctors, nurses, and clerks who read medical records and call doctors to question them, sometimes in extreme detail, about their patients. These callers demand information about even the most sensitive psychiatric history. All the information they obtain goes into their vast computer databases.

While all these reasons to access *your* medical records may each be legitimate and appropriate, some of which are even highly desirable, the sum total is the potential for very widespread dissemination of your personal information and a near total destruction of the concept of privacy. This is true even when every person and agency is abiding by all the rules and is acting completely ethically and within the law.

The Fourth Amendment of the Bill of Rights has as its essential purpose the guarantee of a zone of privacy for every citizen, a right increasingly established in the courts as well. In addition there are privileges firmly established in common law and legal precedent—the nearly inviolable privilege of confidentiality of all communications between husband and wife, doctor and patient, lawyer and client, and religious mentor and those they hear in confidence. Recently the privilege was extended to accountants and clients to some degree.

There are many rules and regulations on both federal and state levels pertaining to privacy, use of many kinds of records, and so on. These laws are under examination now and there is heated debate as to whether to increase privacy protection or to ease it for law enforcement and other purposes. Congress has been considering legislation for some time. (Documents regarding privacy can be downloaded from the Health and Human Services website—http://www.hhs.gov—and can serve as a starting point for those who want to pursue this further.) I believe that there is inadequate regulation to require that you be informed any time any agency or person has legally gained access to your information.

Patients may not realize that the medical record maintained by a doctor or hospital is the property of the doctor or hospital. Thus if the doctor or hospital releases information in your medical record, they could be seen as exercising control of their property. However, is not the *information* in the record *your* property? I feel strongly that it is, but it is not that clear in the law. In practice, there are ethical and written rules that prohibit release of your personal information without your consent under most circumstances. Also, if you are informed of a subpoena to access your records you can take legal action to attempt to block that access, but obviously that is a cumbersome and daunting task. Few people would be able to take such steps to preserve their privacy, unless perhaps the request for records was for a criminal investigation. However, since the law is somewhat muddled as to the requirement to notify you when your information is being released, you may not always have the option to attempt to preserve your privacy.

Insurance companies may access a record only if the patient has signed a release allowing it. Your privacy may not be invaded without your consent, but once you give consent you surrender your right to privacy of the information you released. However, under the law, and by common sense, consent is valid only if it is given freely without coercion. Consent that is coerced—obtained under threat of harm—is prohibited. The police cannot beat a confession out of you, your employer cannot force you to consent to an inappropriate request by threatening to fire you if you refuse, someone cannot blackmail you into something or extort money from you by a threat of disclosure of embarrassing material about you. This is one of the freedoms that generations of Americans have shed blood to defend.

What might be termed an *induced* consent is that which is not coerced by direct force or threat, but it is consent that is obtained by imposing a condition on its refusal. In health care, you cannot obtain health insurance without signing a release for the insurance company to obtain any and all information it deems necessary to sell insurance to you and to administer it after you become a policy holder. You voluntarily give consent, but do you really? Very few Americans can afford health care without insurance. The plight of the 42 million uninsured makes that quite clear. You are forced to choose between surrendering your privacy, a right deeply imbedded in the foundations of our democracy and in the ethics of most of us, or forgo the insurance coverage and thus possibly endanger your health. *Thus, your consent is not truly voluntary but is induced by conditions over which you have no practical control.* There is a trend in the courts that is moving toward extending the concept of coerced consent to include such induced consent, but it is far from well developed.

I believe quite strongly that the induced consent concept applies across many aspects of health care and I also believe that it should be held as a *defective* consent. If the judicial trend could be extended to find that the consents in health care insurance are induced consents and if they decide that such consents cannot be enforced, the result will be havoc in health care and in many other fields. The thirty-four years I have spent guarding the most intimate secrets of a legion of patients have always convinced me that privacy is invaluable and worth a very high cost in inconvenience and inefficiency for administrators. I further believe that many of the ways insurers use your private information are misdirected and detrimental, such as in denial of services based on cost, entering your information into databases, and other issues we have been discussing. In the last chapter of this book I describe a new way to provide health insurance that I feel would better preserve privacy and obviate the need for most insurance company access to your records.

Why do I care so much and why should you? In my interviews for my research, some people told me that they do not care who knows what about them. That is fine, that is completely their right, but it must be *their* choice, no one else's.

My first concern is that one of the most important reasons we declared independence in 1776 was to preserve *inalienable* rights and to establish that governments derive "their just powers from the consent of the governed." A right is not something applied when convenient and then forgotten when there is a conflicting desire. We must preserve our fundamental rights at all times with all our vigor, even when seemingly unimportant, or we will lose them. Expediency and claims of necessity, even if important, are not reasons enough to violate those rights that keep our country free and strong.

I believe that today the right to privacy is being eroded slowly but surely across the breadth of our society. Computers amass and connect information about every citizen when there is almost any financial transaction. Most information in computers is not well protected and that which is secure now is unlikely to remain so. Every successful computer security measure is defeated by a more successful computer expert or hacker (the anonymous computer experts who delight in invading other people's computers for fun or for illegal profit). The Internet is among the least secure computer uses. As the country becomes increasingly dependent on the Internet for banking, commerce, information, communication, and record-keeping, privacy issues must be addressed, but so far efforts and laws have been very limited. The *New York Times* reported in a front-page article on August 16, 1998, "Some of the largest commercial sites on the World Wide Web [the Internet] have agreed to feed information about their customers' reading, shopping and entertainment habits into a system developed by a Massachusetts company that is already tracking the moves of more than 30 million Internet users, recording where they go and what they read, often without the users' knowledge."[1] The article goes on to describe both how this method could help consumers by targeting ads to their interests and how it raises critical privacy issues. While this particular service says it will avoid health related information and will not keep names, the database and others like it could easily be used or abused to identify the people tracked and to use the information about them for purposes that may not be so benign.

Spy devices, such as incredibly small and powerful cameras and listening devices, can now be placed anywhere, and the news media frequently reports new applications. Satellite cameras high above the earth have such remarkable resolution (the degree of detail a camera can record) that they can read a document over your shoulder as you recline on the chaise lounge in your backyard. EZ Pass is a small transmitter attached to your windshield that registers you as you pass by a tollbooth at slow speed and charges your account later. These devices create a computer record of every bridge, tunnel, and highway that you pass through, which direction and at what time. This information will allow your movements to be tracked by law enforcement and perhaps others. Global Positioning Satellites (GPSs) orbit the earth and new electronic devices use their transmissions to pinpoint your exact location. This can help you find your way, and can also be hooked up to cellular telephones to provide you with access to emergency services wherever you are. Your GPS gadget will guide you when you travel or allow rescuers to find you quickly, but it also allows you to be located for someone else's purpose and it creates another record of your travels. These electronic wonders add convenience and safety, but they also put more of your life history out of your control.

Corporations are consolidating into ever-larger mergers and alliances, further allowing concentration of computer databases in fewer and fewer hands. In the 1972 film *The Anderson Tapes,* Sean Connery portrays an ex-convict who plans and carries out a complicated holdup and is recorded on many different surveillance cameras and recordings made by the FBI and many other agencies, all observing him coincidentally to their own investigations. In the 1974 film *The Conversation,* director Francis Ford Coppola explores the privacy implications of the lead character's surveillance activities. Both films paint a disturbing picture of the potential of surveillance equipment to penetrate and disrupt our lives, and that was when that equipment was very primitive compared to today's extraordinary technology. Who knows what even more amazing developments will undoubtedly occur in the exponential growth of electronic capability?

Why does this matter? Information is power. The information industry has replaced manufacturing as the mainstay of the American economy for that very reason. A government or corporation that knows everything about you has incredible power if it chooses to use that knowledge abusively, even if we make it illegal to do so. George Orwell's famous book *1984* depicted a future totalitarian society where the government maintained its power over every citizen by surveillance so widespread and complete that no one could escape it. Today's technology surpasses even what Orwell predicted. Only time will tell if it is used for the dismal purposes of which he warned. Imagine if Hitler or Stalin had had today's technology at their disposal.

Is all this theoretical? Let us consider practical ways that you might be affected. We will discuss legal uses of information first. There are many laws and regulations that govern use of information and, as we noted, Congress is debating the issues now. An example of legal invasion of privacy that we all experience is telemarketing. Your home is your castle and you should be entitled to be free of intrusion for commercial reasons as well as any other. You choose to allow others access via the telephone, but you expect that access to be for your benefit. Telemarketing is a legal intrusion on your use of a telephone—calls by sellers attempting to sell you something by calling you at home. It is different than junk mail. You can choose not to open junk mail and just throw it away, but you must answer your telephone, which is then in effect an induced consent. To avoid telemarketing you must either not answer your telephone or get an unlisted number, thus isolating yourself, or screen every call, which is very inconvenient and time-consuming. Laws give you the option to decline telemarketing, but in practice that seldom works, as I can attest from personal experience. I have repeatedly exercised my rights under the laws, but I continue to receive as many as three or four calls a day, usually at the dinner hour or as late as 9:30 P.M. I have written to every agency that is supposed to take me off lists but to no avail. Therefore, while there are legally prescribed remedies, they are sometimes useless. Telemarketing is an annoyance and time waster and the issue is complicated by freedom of speech considerations, but the principles it illustrates related to invasion of your personal life are extremely important. Legal remedies to protect privacy are often cumbersome, impractical, or ineffective.

An example of legal invasion of your privacy in the medical area is the application for any insurance where a health history and/or exam is required. Your consent is induced as you can get the insurance only by releasing your information. Any medical history obtained in a life insurance application is entered into a central databank shared by the insurance companies called the MIB (Medical Information Bureau) that is then accessible to every other insurance company. It is very difficult to successfully expunge erroneous information, if you even know it is in your file, to which you have very limited access. You are essentially branded for life. If you have something in your history that might make you a poor risk, even in error, you may find yourself shut out from insurance thereafter. Every computer holding information about you is another resource for those seeking your information legally or illegally.

Another major potential for problems is genetic testing. You can now be tested for the presence of genes that indicate you are at high risk for some types of breast cancer, ovarian cancer, colon cancer, Alzheimer's disease, and Huntington's chorea (the degenerative neurological disease that killed singer Woody Guthrie). These genes do not say you have or definitely will have the disease, only that you are at greater risk. Yet knowledge of these genetic findings could be used to deny you a job or insurance or could affect how people feel about you and relate to you. Another example of the impact of uncertainty about privacy is that women at very high risk of ovarian or breast cancer who may want to consider drastic surgical preventive efforts (prophylactic removal of breasts or ovaries) may fear to get the tests necessary if others might know about it. Managed care companies gather information so assiduously that they may begin to databank genetic information as it becomes available in the course of monitoring their subscribers. While it should not be, currently such specific information as test *results* might be in their databanks if discovered through chart review or questioning your doctor, and the fact that you *had* a test certainly would be. As insurers and the government take on "managing" your care more and more, how far might they go?

Genetic testing promises major advances in combating disease, but it also raises very important ethical issues. An example of the potential and frightening extreme of misuse of genetic information may be a 1994 law of the People's Republic of China, as reported in the *New York Times*.[2] A section of this law mandates genetic counseling, but it also directs that doctors "take steps" such as sterilization or long-term contraception to "prevent childbearing." It is not yet clear, according to the article, just how this law is being applied or enforced, but its very existence raises the specter of the eugenics programs of Hitler's regime in Germany. Eugenics is the attempt to improve populations by controlling genetic characteristics. This is good for making better wheat but very wrong when applied to humans, other than the sensible genetic counseling that occurs today so that parents know the risk for children of genetic diseases they are known to carry. The Nazis killed those people they thought inferior to avoid "pollution" of their "master race." Americans abhor such practices and our Constitution and laws seem a powerful bulwark against such extremes, but we cannot evade the implications of emerging technologies. Democracy succeeds only by the constant vigilance of the people. If we stop looking and caring, harmful changes may occur before we know it.

Though I have many serious reservations about the currently legal uses of health information, let us now consider what few people would disagree is quite serious, the illegal abuse of information. Once information is out of your control, you must depend on the kindness and honesty of strangers to use it legally and ethically. If someone chooses to violate rules and regulations and access your information, which is extremely easy to do and frequently undetectable, you are at their mercy and you seldom even know it. Criminal uses of social security numbers and credit card numbers have soared, according to a recent Government Accounting Office report.[3] Other abuses may be subtler. State and federal laws prohibit discrimination based on disability. Your employer is supposed to simply monitor your benefits, but if he learns from your benefits records that you have had an anti-AIDS drug prescribed, you might find yourself ostracized or fired. A middle-level manager at a Pennsylvania company suffered this problem; while he was kept on the job, the suffering from his illness was compounded by the cruel treatment from his boss and coworkers.[4] The same could happen to people with breast cancer, psychiatric problems, and many other conditions.

Celebrities are particularly good targets for snoopers. For example, singer Tammy Wynette tried to preserve her privacy when she checked into a prestigious Pittsburgh hospital. Shortly after, her entire medical story was on the front page of the *National Enquirer*, highly exaggerated and distorted, but based on her actual record. It had been accessed by a hospital employee and the information sold to the *Enquirer*.[5]

There are many other examples involving improper or illegal penetration of medical records: hospital employees who sold printouts of information to sales representatives of managed care companies; a convicted child rapist who accessed a thousand confidential files and made scores of calls to teenage girls asking for dates; a thirteen-year-old girl who used an emergency room computer to get names and telephone numbers of seven patients whom she then called and frightened severely by telling them, falsely, that they had AIDS; and the Harvard Community Health Plan, a prestigious Boston HMO, which posted many patients' sensitive psychiatric files in on-line patient records which were available to many people totally unconnected with those cases (they subsequently improved their procedures).[6]

These stories simply illustrate how easy it is to gain access to information and the harmful effects loss of privacy can have. There are countless other ways you could be adversely affected if your information is misused. Once out of your control, anything can happen.

The 1996 Health Care Portability and Accountability Act (the Kennedy-Kassebaum bill described previously) included the provision to establish a national health identification card. *U.S. News and World Report* recently published an interview with Robert Gellman, a Washington, D.C., privacy consultant who serves on the Department of Health and Human Services committee working on the health ID card.[7] He expressed serious concerns. He noted that a national identifier would help some research, might improve coordination of a patient's care, and perhaps reduce costs and increase administrative efficiency, but it would cost at least $10 billion to implement. He stated,

> My real concern is that a health ID would become a national ID overnight. An incredible number of people would have access to this number—your doctor, dentist, pharmacy, insurance company, employer, and your employer's health plan, your bank, credit bureaus, the police, and government agencies like the IRS, welfare, and immigration. You might not want your employer to know you are seeing a psychiatrist or that your child has spina bifida [a birth defect that causes permanent paralysis below the waist], which could drive up the cost of the company health plan. The notion that the ID would be just for health purposes is absurd.[8]

Gellman was referring to the ID card, but the above description applies to much of the way your information is handled even if it is not as easily accessed as it would be with a single identifier. He notes that "All members of the European Union [the new coalition of most of the major European countries] have comprehensive privacy laws saying records collected for one purpose can't be used for another. *Some* [italics added] of these concerns would be allayed if we had similar laws."[9] He voted against the proposal within his committee but was in the minority. Even without a national identifier, databases are being combined or connected anyway by mergers and cooperative agreements between the companies that maintain them.

Another expert, Georgetown University law professor Lawrence Gostin, says that, sadly, privacy has disappeared. He argues, however, "There are trade-offs between privacy and the goods society gets from medicine. And information is the life's blood of the modern health-care system. The public should get reasonable assurances that when their personal information is collected, the health-care system will treat it with respect, store it securely, and disclose it only for important health purposes."[10]

Hospital records are easily accessed by many people, even with improving security measures, and Medicare is gathering increasingly large volumes of data about millions of Americans. Managed care is not the only problem, but it is among the worst. Managed care companies know what doctors you have seen, what your diagnoses are, what treatments you have received (and continue to receive), and sometimes even your most private secrets. The powerful profit motive inherent in for-profit managed care may lead them to rationalize uses of your information that you may well find distressing. The list of assaults on your personal information seems endless.

In a fascinating book called *Why Things Bite Back: Technology and the Revenge of Unintended Consequences,* Edward Tenner shows in many examples how new technologies of real value to us nevertheless can result in totally unexpected adverse consequences.[11] He does not discuss the impact of technology on privacy, but what we have discussed here is a perfect example of how social policy and even very desirable technology can pose unexpected danger. I use EZ Pass and I would love to have a GPS gadget. I purchase insurance and do all the other things we have been discussing. While some things, like telemarketing, are completely unacceptable to me, I certainly feel strongly that we can never go back to a noncomputerized world. My concern is how we preserve the value of the new developments without surrendering our most precious rights. I believe that no technology, no social policy, no political philosophy is worth surrendering the foundations of our freedom. I would choose freedom in a cave over the world of *1984.* We do not have to make that choice. We can find solutions that will preserve both our rights and our technology if we begin with the same conviction to freedom that drove our founding fathers (and mothers) to create the freest and greatest country in history.

However, if we allow the current trend toward consolidation of information and power into fewer and fewer hands to continue unchecked and uncontrolled, then we should all fear for the future of our democracy. If we are to fight back, we must all decide how much control of our lives we want to surrender. Those of us who believe that privacy is a right worth defending should speak up, as I am doing now. Call your congressperson and demand strict new laws, including the kinds used in Europe. We as individuals have to struggle doubly hard against opposing forces that are rich and powerful. To do nothing allows others to win by default. Americans must never forget that one consequence of our democracy is that we get the government we ask for. Only by working together can ordinary people compete against those whose power and wealth have influence in Congress.

It is not too late, but there is not much time left before the loss of privacy becomes irreversible. In health care, as the above discussion suggests, the problem cannot readily be dealt with by tinkering here and there. I believe that only substantial changes, such as I suggest in my proposals in the last chapter, will succeed.

NOTES

1. Saul Hansell, "Big Websites to Track Steps of Their Users," *New York Times*, August 16, 1998, 1, 24.
2. Elizabeth Rosenthal, "Scientists Debate China's Law on Sterilizing the Carriers of Genetic Defects," *New York Times*, August 16, 1998, 14.
3. "Criminal Use of ID Information Reported on the Rise," *Physicians Financial News*, August 15, 1998, 14.
4. John Riley, "Open Secrets," *Newsday*, March 31, 1996, A5.
5. Ibid.
6. Ibid., p. 32.
7. "Medical ID Plan Stirs Fears of Big Brother," *U.S. News & World Report* (August 3, 1998): 62.
8. Ibid.
9. Ibid.
10. Arthur Allen, "Medical Privacy? Forget It!" *Medical Economics*, (May 11, 1998): 157.
11. Edward Tenner, *Why Things Bite Back* (New York: Alfred A. Knopf, 1996).

9

Does Managed Care Fulfill Its Promise to Preserve Quality of Care While Reducing Cost?

Managed care was conceived to improve care by managing it better than doctors could do when left to their own devices. Has it succeeded?

Managed care companies make many promises. Their advertisements, brochures, and publications suggest that they can deliver *high*-quality care at *low* prices and reasonably prompt service. That would be nice if true, but:

- You cannot have quality when you refuse to pay for it.
- The prices *seem* lower than they would have been in traditional insurance, but only because the service delivered is reduced.
- Requests for many services may be delayed by denials and prolonged periods of appeal, sometimes until it is too late to do any good, as George Anders describes in *Health against Wealth.*

What is quality? Quality care is that delivered by the Good Doctor I have described in chapter 2. How do you measure quality? You can't. As Dean Ornish recently quoted a colleague, *not everything that counts can be counted.*

Managed care has spawned whole new industries that try to measure and calculate quality, cost-effectiveness, customer satisfaction (there are no more patients, just "customers" and "clients" who go to "providers"), and anything else they can put a ruler against, all in an attempt to justify managed care.

There is truth and there is what can be measured. A famous principle in quantum physics says that the act of studying something changes it. If you shine a light on an object so that you can measure the object's temperature, you will record a slightly higher temperature than the object really is because the light will have warmed it slightly. Likewise, how you ask a question influences the answer. Pollsters know how to do polls that are accurate, but they also know how to conduct a poll to get the outcome they want. For example, pollsters know that people often answer in the way they think the questioner wants to hear. It is easy to capitalize on that tendency by asking the right questions. "We are very proud of our widgets. Do you like them, too?" Polling and research should search for truth, but what is truth? Truth may be different from what you can measure, which will differ from what you *choose* to measure, which will differ from how you choose to interpret and describe what you have measured. Suppose you are an HMO and want to prove that your customers are satisfied with your service. The customers are actually very unhappy with the HMO because of all the things we have been discussing. You want your HMO to sound loved. How to do that? First, you want to avoid any questions that might pertain to treatment when they are ill or to their choice of doctor or to privacy issues and so on. Instead, you would want to concentrate on the lack of paperwork, immunizations, well-baby checkups, the huge number of doctors on the panel, those nice newsletters you send out, and the lollipops for kids on every visit.

You would then carefully couch your questions. For example, you could ask:

Which do you prefer?

a. Your old insurance where you could see the doctor of your choice, no one butted into your business, and you could get what you need, or,
b. Our insurance where you can only see our doctors, we decide what is good for you and how much we want to allow you to have, and, oh yes, we can read your most personal and intimate information that you thought was private.

What business that expects to remain viable would ask the question that way?

Instead, you might ask it the same way, but you add to (b), "Our insurance is $10 less per month." Then you might actually get some takers for answer (b). But even then the risks are high. But if you ask a much more general question: "Of all the choices your employer gave you, do you like ours the best?" You may well receive a reply that shows your HMO in a very positive light.

When you publish the survey in your full-color brochure, the reader will not know that the employer only offered one plan, or only gave the respondents a choice of a few HMOs. The yes answer meant not that those asked liked their plan, only that it was the best of a bad lot. But if two-thirds (67 percent) of the respondents said, "Yeah, I guess so," and one quarter (25 percent) said, "Yeah, its better than the other plan, but [rest of answer cut off]," your HMO can then brag that you have a "92 percent approval rating in a customer satisfaction survey!"

This is no exaggeration. For some people this is the science of polling—how to ask questions to get the answer you want. The same knowledge *can* be used to try to *avoid* influencing the answer and to ensure reasonable accuracy when real information is needed. You can be sure that a politician's or a corporation's *private* polls are done in the most accurate way and that the polls that are publicized are done in the manipulative way.

Major pollsters like Gallup maintain high standards; nevertheless, their clients or others may misuse or misstate their results despite strict rules against it. Gallup recently chastised a customer who claimed a high satisfaction rate but failed to note that the survey only included successful subjects. Obviously, if you confine your poll only to people with good results, your product will sound great.

Another part of the measurement industry is "quality assessment." Managed care maintains that it preserves the quality of care at a low price. What is "quality of care"?

Managed care applied industrial production methods such as TQM (Total Quality Measurement) or CQI (Continuous Quality Improvement) which were developed to improve heavy manufacturing, like autos and steel.[1] These techniques measure assembly lines, like car production, in detailed ways that allow new kinds of mathematical analysis and management techniques to improve efficiency and productivity. When doctors tried to argue that people were not machines on an assembly line, they were derided as old-fashioned. Big corporate buyers of managed care insurance loved the use of management tools that they used in their own businesses.[2]

You can count only what you can measure. You can measure only what is recorded. The head of one of the largest HMOs often said, "It doesn't count if you can't count it."[3] In other words, it does not matter what a doctor *does*, it only matters what is *recorded* and if it is something the HMO wants to count. For example, a managed care nurse reviewed the chart of a clinic patient in a managed care plan I had seen. This patient was a very strict observer of his religion and his religious beliefs meant that the *only* woman he had had sexual relations with was his wife and that he would *never* disrobe in public to sunbathe. I had helped this patient solve some very serious medical problems, but the reviewer took no note of that and rated the chart to be of poor quality because I had not advised this patient to wear a sunblocker and get an HIV test to look for AIDS exposure, two preventive measures that must have been on her checklist. She ignored the care of actual diseases and applied ordinarily reasonable advice by rote to a patient who had no need of it.

The HMOs use the it-only-counts-if-we-can-count-it method in several ways that George Anders describes very effectively in his book. First, they use this excuse to set up quality guidelines and measurements that monitor only simple, easy-to-do items such as those I just described because they claim everything else is too complex to make any meaningful measurements. Second, they use the same approach with top teaching hospitals. Major teaching centers cost more because they attract the most difficult patients, they have the best and most expensive facilities and tools, they are the cauldrons that create medical advances, and they attract staff who do research and teaching as well as patient care. The very qualities that distinguish teaching centers from smaller, stand-alone hospitals, such as the expenses for teaching medical students, research, laboratories and clinics to address diseases and problems beyond the scope of the smaller facilities, are not adequately reflected in the measures managed care uses to decide reimbursement levels. Thus, these centers are undergoing financial strain because they are reimbursed close to the same rates as the smaller hospitals, which do not have the same expenses. In this case, the managed care companies can argue that it is not their responsibility to fund the additional costs of teaching centers and that society should find alternative ways. That may be a valid point of view, but it is contrary to the long-established traditional function that health insurance played in the past and politically it may be difficult to achieve. The public will pay for teaching centers one way or another—either as higher taxes for public funding or as higher premiums if managed care takes on the responsibility—or lose invaluable resources that have helped make American medicine as good as it is. While one might say that social good is not the business of business, I strongly disagree. We do not want corporations dictating social policy, but just as individuals contribute for the good of others might not business share some of their profits?

Such contributions from profits would not increase prices but would improve the social environment in which business must operate.

A major source of managed care quality control and enhancement efforts is the National Committee for Quality Assurance (NCQA), a private, nonprofit organization headed by a very large, distinguished panel of experts in managed care and related fields. The panelists include experts on quality measurement and managed care and representatives from employers, corporations, health plans, universities, consumer and labor organizations, and organized medicine. An NCQA publication for consumers on its website* includes this statement: "NCQA's mission is to provide information that enables purchasers and consumers of managed health care to distinguish among plans based on quality and value, thereby allowing them to make more informed health care purchasing decisions. This will encourage plans to compete on quality and value, rather than on price and provider network alone."[4]

The NCQA performs evaluations for accreditation and to gauge performance of health plans. For accreditation, it judges the plan on NCQA's standards covering quality management and improvement (what does the plan do to monitor and enhance quality of care and delivery of its services); does the plan carefully check and recheck the credentials of its doctors and other professionals; does it keep members well informed about their rights under the plan and how best to use it; does it respond to member satisfaction ratings; does it perform a variety of preventive health services; is the plan reasonable in meeting members' needs and providing services; does it maintain good medical records; and a variety of other, related factors.

The NCQA monitors plans' performance primarily based on the Health Plan Employer Data and Information Set (HEDIS®). HEDIS is a set of more than fifty performance measures† designed to give a comprehensive view of the care delivered by the plans. Some examples of these measures include advising smokers to quit; eye exams for people with diabetes; cervical cancer screening; immunizations; the rate of smokers who quit; screening for various diseases; whether treatment for depression is being maintained; the availability of doctors and dentists; satisfaction ratings by members; qualifications of doctors;

---

*NCQA's website, a helpful source to learn more about the organization and its methods, is found at http://www.ncqa.org.

†A list of these measures is found at http://www.ncqa.org/news/hedismeas.htm, August 16, 1998.

how well the plan is carrying out quality assessment; utilization management; risk management; and more in the same vein.

These are all reasonable things to measure and to the degree that managed care helps doctors improve performance in preventive medicine, following up on patient care, keeping good records, and the like, it contributes toward its goal of improving quality of care. However, a careful review of the HEDIS criteria will demonstrate that, as both Linda Peeno observed in her direct experience and George Anders found from his extensive research, managed care does little or nothing to measure the performance of care of acute and serious illness. I would add that my own studies of the doctor-patient relationship lead me to believe that all these measures also fail to assess the quality of the vitally important relationship between doctor and patient.

Many aspects of medical care are difficult to measure and document. Take rheumatoid arthritis, for example. One of my subspecialties is rheumatology (the care of arthritis and related diseases). Rheumatoid arthritis is a difficult disease to study. There are no specific diagnostic tests; diagnosis is made on a clinical impression based on a broad set of clues in the history, the physical exam, the laboratory, and X-rays and MRI scans (scans using magnetic fields and computers to give remarkably detailed images of internal body parts). The best way to judge results of most treatment is to obtain results that can be measured and tabulated. In rheumatoid arthritis there are practically none.

We can follow trends in some lab tests but one of the main monitoring measures is how many joints are red and painful and how long stiffness lasts in the morning. These are highly subjective observations for both the patient and the doctor. This means that moods, hopes, and beliefs can easily influence the accuracy of these observations. Thus, the true measure of rheumatoid arthritis is the clinical sense gained by frequent visits, time spent listening to and advising the patient, and knowing him or her as a whole person.

Perhaps most important, HMOs do not measure the value that patients feel when they know they have a real doctor they can trust and turn to when in need. HMOs do not measure quality, but only quantifiable results.

NOTES

1. George Anders, *Health against Wealth, HMOs and the Breakdown of Medical Trust* (New York: Houghton Mifflin, 1996).

2. Ibid.

3. Ibid.

4. "National Committee for Quality Assurance: An Overview," http://www.ncqa.org/overview3.htm, August 16, 1998.

10

How Medicine Is Affected by Legal and Ethical Trends in Practice

There are many ways in which legal and ethical issues related to managed care and other aspects of medicine influence medical care.

HOW MANAGED CARE AFFECTS WHAT DOCTORS MAY TELL PATIENTS

Managed care companies not only insist on deciding to what you are entitled, they even want to control what you know.

Informed consent, as we discussed in chapter 2, is a moral, professional, and legal necessity in any doctor-patient interaction. Operating on a competent patient without the consent of that patient is a battery, which Webster's dictionary defines as the "unlawful use of force" on a person. A consent that is obtained without a reasonable degree of understanding by the person asked to sign it is not a true consent. Consent applies to all medical care, not just the obvious case of surgery or some other invasive procedure.

Managed care places the physician in many ethically untenable positions, many of which we have already discussed:

- serving two masters
- fee splitting
- being forced to choose between the needs of the patient and the doctor's own financial interest

- cutting funding so close to the bone that there is no room for backup safety measures and no flexibility to allow for all the individual variations to which each person is prone
- allowing inadequate time with patients
- limiting payments to treatments the insurer chooses regardless of the judgment of the doctor
- substituting a lesser trained practitioner (e.g., physician's assistant) for a physician

To these we can add another: lack of adequate informed consent. Managed care companies restrict doctors from informing patients in several ways.

Some companies have actual, specific "gag" rules written into their contract with the doctor that specifically prohibit the doctor from criticizing the HMO. In such cases, the doctor may not reveal what the HMO calls "proprietary" information, which includes most of the methods HMOs use to pay doctors, the financial incentives or penalties that influence how the doctor practices. Some contracts have even said the doctor should not advise the patient of treatments, specialists, etc., that the doctor may feel are indicated but that the HMO does not approve. For example, if a doctor feels you need an operation, hospital admission, or various kinds of tests, he first has to get approval from the HMO. If the HMO declines the request, the more restrictive gag rules would prohibit the doctor from even telling the patient about what he would have recommended. The patient is not to be told that the doctor makes more money if less is done.

Even when there is no explicit gag clause, there is unwritten pressure to comply anyway because the HMO holds the doctor's livelihood in its hands.

This is not an idle threat—it has happened. Consider the case of a dermatologist who requested approval from the patient's HMO to remove some benign-looking scalp lesions and to send them to pathology for review. The HMO approved the surgery but refused to approve the pathology, which would examine the tissue under the microscope to look for signs of cancer.[1]

The dermatologist argued as best he could that the type of lesion he was removing *could* be malignant, though admittedly such cases were rare. The HMO was adamant. The dermatologist felt so strongly about it that he paid for the pathology himself and informed the patient of the disagreement. The dermatologist's malpractice insurance carrier advised him to write a letter to the HMO and to the local

No matter how benign-looking a lesion may be, with very few exceptions, there is always a risk of a malignancy (cancer). In my opinion, it is gross negligence to fail to send a specimen to pathology in all but the few cases where the lesion is extremely small and of the type that are never serious, and those are very few.

As an example, virtually every one of us has at least a few small fatty tumors, called lipomas. They are at most annoying and need never be removed for any reason other than the patient's choice, except in those few cases where they feel abnormal or change more quickly than usual. If they are removed, they should always be sent to pathology. An HMO might argue that this is a waste of money. It is not.

A physician friend of mine saw two patients in one week who had lipomas removed that on pathology examination proved *malignant!* Thanks to his thoroughness, both patients should do well. He did not just assume that the lipomas were benign. He ordered the biopsy and the pathology exams.

Had he not done so, had he not had the pathology report to make the correct diagnosis, both patients might have progressed to a state that was incurable, but his approach allowed early, definitive, curative treatment. (This does *not* mean that if you find such a lump on yourself you should be frightened—they are very rarely cancerous! Let your doctor check it for you.)

medical society, which he did. He then received a letter back from the HMO telling him that he had not behaved in a "collegial mode with us in this matter." They claimed that their decision was based on "sound science" and that there should be "mutual trust and understanding of our respective roles." He was warned that this correspondence was being entered in his "Quality Management File."

This terminology is one of many euphemistic ways to warn physicians that if they do not shape up, they will be shipped out. Obviously, the dermatologist cannot assume the cost of every patient's pathology tests. Even worse, what happens if the HMO declines to pay for even more expensive tests? The doctor is placed in a painful dilemma—ignore what he knows is proper medical practice, go broke trying to compensate for the HMO's failure to provide fair coverage, or tell the patient that even though the HMO won't pay for that, he strongly urges that it be done.

Such conflicts of interest, about which patients are not informed, can take other forms. Let me pose a hypothetical extreme case to illustrate the point. Suppose you develop liver disease. You are in a global capitated plan, which means that the medical group holding your contract is responsible for the entire cost of your care, no matter what. They have assumed the full financial risk of their assigned pool of insureds. Global capitation can be highly profitable, but that advantage is balanced by much higher financial risk. The plan is counting on its members remaining well.

But in your case the condition worsens. The doctors in the medical group meet to discuss your case. The consensus is that you are a reasonable candidate for a liver transplant. Now they are faced with a difficult choice. Do they offer you a liver transplant that could save your life? If they do, it may cost *them* as much as hundreds of thousands of dollars and seriously impair their financial condition. *You* are their worst nightmare.

Do they advise you of the option? Do they delay long enough that it becomes a moot point—you have become too sick to do the operation? Delay is a favorite tactic of cost-cutters. Not only do they receive the "float"—continuing to collect interest on moneys delayed in disbursement—but sometimes the patient dies before they have to do anything.

The idea of insurance is that we all pay in to a common pool, hoping we will never need the benefits, but, if we do, with the fair expectation that we will get the help we paid for. When managed care creates a situation in which *your* care comes right out of the pocket of someone else, who pays the price—you or them? Remember that *they* have the power. In the traditional indemnity insurance the pool was very large and could absorb the exceptional high-cost case, but a medical group holding a capitation contract does not have the resources or capitalization to do so.

If you are in a noncapitated HMO, remember the young HMO medical director who revealed the 10 percent bonus. That means if *your* doctor recommends a liver transplant, finding a reason to reject that $300,000 operation could be worth $30,000 to *their* medical director.

Consider another hypothetical example of a simpler situation. You consult your doctor about a kidney problem. He determines that you need a kidney X-ray called an IVP. He asks you if you are allergic to shellfish. You are a little puzzled as you tell him how you get hives whenever you eat shrimp. The last time you ate them you developed shortness of breath and felt wheezes.

He tells you that shrimp are high in iodine and thus you might be allergic to iodine, which is an ingredient of the contrast material used intravenously to make your kidneys stand out on the X-ray. He tells you that there is a risk of a life-threatening reaction, but he is going to give you some corticosteroids before the procedure to block the reaction. You feel well informed.

You are reassured, go through with the test, have a severe reaction, and barely survive. Then you find out that there were two alternatives. The particular information needed could have been obtained by an MRI without any iodine dye, but an MRI is seven times more expensive than the IVP. Or, you learn, the IVP could have been done with a new contrast material that is iodine-free, specifically developed for people allergic to iodine, but that the new type is ten times more expensive than the iodine type.

You were not informed that you were offered a riskier choice—in fact, you were not even told you had a choice—and you certainly were not informed that your treatment was decided on cost rather than safety.

I believe that proper informed consent means telling the patient *all* the available options and the benefits and risks of each, as best the physician knows. I always advise patients of any controversy about the test or the treatment if I am aware of differing opinions. I tell the patient what I would recommend, but I try to make sure the patient knows the whole spectrum of belief on the issue, as far as I know about it.

Patients *should* be advised of costs. First, the patient will likely have to pay some portion of the cost and we should all have a fair say in how we spend our own money. Second, since almost all care is paid for at least partly by shared funds, we should all, patient and doctor, be as prudent as we can be in spending money wisely. That is quite different from making secret decisions purely for profit. When managed care puts so much pressure on its case reviewers, as Linda Peeno described, and rewards them with strong financial incentives to deny care, they may bow to the pressures and overlook the welfare of the patients.

HOW MANAGED CARE AVOIDS LEGAL RESPONSIBILITY FOR ITS ACTIONS

"Malpractice" means either negligence or the commission of an error so egregious that a reasonably trained and careful individual would not have committed it. Unfortunately, our legal brethren have contorted this rather straightforward principle to create a new industry, one highly profitable to them. They have transformed malpractice from negligence into compensation for unfortunate outcomes. We are all aware of the tremendous burden this imposes on the system.

Many adverse outcomes are due to circumstances medicine's current level of knowledge cannot control:

- Treatments do not work every time, even when done properly. For example, a cancer specialist starts a patient on a promising new treatment for breast cancer but in this case it fails and the cancer progresses.
- Diagnoses are not always correct even when the diagnostic process was entirely appropriate. Scans of the abdomen may indicate strongly that a patient's pain is due to a malignant tumor and surgery is indicated. The patient undergoes a major operation, but pathology on the removed mass shows that it was benign (noncancerous) and was an incidental finding that did not require major surgery.
- Medications properly prescribed do not always work and they sometimes even make the patient worse. Consider a patient with a serious bacterial skin infection. The doctor prescribes an antibiotic, but in this case the bacterial infection is resistant to it and the infection spreads and causes complications. If the patient happens to become allergic to the antibiotic at that point, the reaction can make things worse.
- Operations performed perfectly may fail for reasons beyond the surgeon's control, such as occured in the heart operation I describe a little later in this chapter.
- Babies may be born damaged or defective for reasons having nothing to do with the obstetrician's care. The baby may have had a genetic defect not yet detectable prenatally or a virus infection there was no way to know about.

None of these constitutes malpractice, yet far too frequently malpractice suits are filed over them even though no negligence has occurred. A good lawyer can make *any* reasonable medical treatment or procedure *sound* negligent. Juries may be convinced by an appeal to their empathy for a patient who has suffered and may feel that *someone* should pay for it. They feel that malpractice insurance companies are rich and can well afford it.

Trial lawyers right now are pursuing approximately 120,000 lawsuits against the 738,000 American doctors. Over 40 percent of physicians are sued at least once.[2]

I have never been sued, but I know many superb physicians who have been, all unfairly. The receipt of a subpoena announcing a lawsuit against them is one of the worst experiences they have ever had, even when they knew they were innocent, or were sued by mistake regarding patients they did not even know. (For instance, it would not be unusual in a large city for two different doctors to have the same name, allowing the possibility of a subpoena being served on the wrong person.) I know personally of ten doctors who were sued in cases where they had never seen the patient or where the plaintiff's case was egregiously defective. Most doctors are so driven by the responsibility for someone else's life that they feel compelled to be perfect. A lawsuit is like a blow to their very being and soul. It is also highly disruptive of their practices and their personal life. While malpractice insurance pays the cost of litigation and any losses due to settlement or a lost case, the doctor incurs lost income and other expenses. This is bad enough when the doctor is innocent and even more galling when he has been mistakenly sued.

Even an error is not malpractice. No person can achieve perfection. We must draw a *reasonable* line between an error that any reasonably careful person could make under the real circumstances of everyday life and an error or injury that occurs because the person did not take the care that would be expected of a reasonable person under those circumstances. Acceptable medical practice may be a legal defense, but what is acceptable is so open to debate that it becomes a battle of experts from both sides that often leaves the jury without clear information as to what is acceptable. Juries are not equipped on their own to comprehend the highly technical nature of modern medicine. Juries often decide on their own that, in effect, malpractice payouts are social tools to make a point or to help someone they feel deserves it.

Even beyond the medical world, too many juries are deciding that if there is a bad result, someone should pay—but only if there is someone with enough money to make it worth the lawyer's while. (Bars are held responsible for drunk drivers' actions and even lawyers must themselves purchase "malpractice" insurance in case they lose a case and their client needs someone to blame.) Malpractice suits are based on contingency fees, which means the lawyer collects a fee only if the lawsuit is won. This allows even the poorest plaintiff to get representation, but only in cases where there is the possibility of a large enough award for the lawyer to take the risk.

True malpractice is deplorable. No doctor should be negligent in the care of patients. It is a sacred trust that brooks no exceptions. However, we all make errors because we are all human. We should not be held to standards of perfection, only to the standard of always doing our best.

In my last year of medical school, I asked one of the heart surgeons if I could observe an open-heart operation. The patient was a fifty-year-old woman whose diseased heart valve was failing. I went to visit her. She was weak, could not function well, and was short of breath with the slightest exertion. Without surgery, she would become progressively more disabled and then die. I was not her doctor, just a student, but she welcomed my visit and shared her feelings. She was a lovely person and I wished her well.

The next day, I scrubbed up and joined the surgeons in the operating room. I had no role other than that of observer. The surgeons were very kind and explained things as they went along. Then they became very quiet. Murmured concerns and low voices telegraphed that something was going wrong. When they could, they explained to me that the patient had a rare condition that weakened the supportive tissue around the valve. This condition was probably the reason for the valve disease in the first place, but it was making the repair impossible. Every stitch they put in pulled away—the weak tissue would not sustain it.

The early heart-lung life support machines of that day were safe only for a limited time and the operation was reaching that limit. The surgeons did not give up. They tried everything that their combined decades of experience had taught them. A procedure that should have taken only a few hours became four, then six, then more. I finally left after nine hours and found out later that they had stayed another hour more. Nothing had worked and the patient did not survive the operation.

As a fourth-year student, this was not the first patient I had seen die, but it is always painful. Even after thirty years, even when it is inevitable and you have done all you can, death is still the hardest part of medicine.

Those surgeons made the correct decision to operate. They were among the most skilled and experienced in the country in one of the world's best hospitals and everything was done according to the highest standards. The patient's condition was simply beyond repair even in the best of hands. In medicine, there is always risk and there are no guarantees.

Today, those surgeons would probably be sued. Had they been negligent, I would testify against them, but they were not and I would demand to be heard in their defense as they certainly performed well above the level of acceptable medical practice.

Doctors must hold themselves to the highest standards *from within.* External threats do not make good doctors. Nevertheless, there is nothing wrong and everything right that we should all be held accountable if we fail in our obligations to uphold the responsibility we have been given.

The public assumes that medicine as a profession is something like a club where members defend each other even when wrong. In my experience, that perception is mostly unfounded, but that distrust has certainly been a factor in the rise in malpractice suits.

Physician malpractice is a serious problem that needs addressing, but unfortunately current attempts at external control backfire because the exaggerated threat of malpractice distorts medical practice and produces defensive medicine, in which excess tests and treatments are ordered in fear of later second-guessing by others if something goes wrong. I believe external threats like malpractice are only marginally effective ways to positively influence doctors' behavior, and the price we pay for malpractice does not justify this small benefit. We certainly need to control poor care by inferior or defective doctors and to compensate injured people in a reasonable way, but today's system does not properly achieve those goals.

Insurance companies that today exercise so much influence over what the doctor does should be held to the same accountability, but they have found a special immunity. For a long time, the companies hid behind a 1974 federal law, the Employee Retirement and Income Security Act (ERISA). This law was not intended for HMOs, but they latched on to it because it allowed some issues related to employee benefit plans to be transferred to federal court. Federal court awards are usually much more limited than those of state courts, which makes suits less lucrative and therefore less likely to find lawyers to bring them to court.[3]

ERISA was designed for consumers' benefit to help regulate pension plans and similar financial instruments. It may be doing that well. While it specifically precludes state action in these cases we are discussing, it leaves HMOs a shield that has not yet been balanced by scrutiny in the federal forum, as this book suggests would be appropriate.

The shifting of malpractice suits to federal courts, where inappropriate jury verdicts are unlikely to be a factor, may well be one step toward improving how we handle all malpractice, but at this point the inability to hold insurers responsible for their effects on patient care is a major concern. In addition, insurers have mostly prevailed in convincing courts that they are only insurers and do not practice medicine, a view I strongly dispute. If a court holds that the insurer was not practicing medicine, the insurer cannot be held liable for malpractice and the plaintiff is limited to seeking to hold only the physicians involved in their care responsible.

In some cases, such as one against an HIP group, described on the local NBC Evening News in New York City on April 28, 1998, the HMO could not be sued for malpractice because it was held to be only an insurer that hired a group of doctors. Even though, as the story implied, the HMO denials might have been responsible for the injury to the child in question, this claim was not allowed to be tested in court; only the doctors were able to be sued.

An insurer's lawyer might also have argued that since the insurer did not stop the patient from getting a denied procedure at his own expense, they did not cause the consequences of the denial. However, as we have noted, few people can afford expensive procedures on their own, so in practical terms the HMO deprived them of the service.

HMOs have steadfastly refused to acknowledge any responsibility for outcomes of the care of their customers. They maintain that they are just insurance companies and that the patient's doctor decides medical care. These strategies have proved an impregnable legal fortress until recently. However, in most cases HMOs still *cannot* be held accountable for the consequences of their policies and actions.[4] They want it both ways. They want to control the care their doctors provide but claim "That's not my job" when problems occur. They want to be immune from the consequences of their own actions and policies. They have heavily lobbied against all attempts at legislation that would make them liable. The repeated refrain against all laws that would limit HMOs' power to control is that they would impair the HMOs' ability to manage costs. They contend that the consumer would be penalized by higher premiums. (Note that the executives never consider reducing *their* multimillion-dollar compensation packages to help the consumers whose needs they claim to protect.) Managed care's immunity from the damage it causes is totally unacceptable.

If HMOs truly believe that their policies are for society's good, they should not hide behind legal loopholes or seek the protection of politicians to whom they have given large contributions. They should be willing to defend their policies openly and at risk of penalty if they cause harm.

A lawsuit is an invaluable societal control mechanism. A sharp blow to the pocketbook gets immediate attention. Consciences—those handy parts of the mind that tell us right from wrong and make us care about which is which—always in short supply in business and industry, seem to have nearly disappeared somewhere between 1960 and 1990. Financial risk has become the surrogate for conscience. Moreover, the creed of the 1990s, as it was in the 1950s, seems to be that the end justifies the means. We need a reasonable level of threat of suit to put some brake on those who lack a conscience and are moved only by threats to their financial health. Making HMOs liable will help force a dramatic and needed shift. Once *they* have to pay for the damage caused by their decisions, they will begin to rethink their methods.

Jethro Lieberman, a lawyer, law professor, and formerly legal affairs editor of *Business Week,* wrote what is probably the first book on the excess litigation problem in America. *The Litigious Society,* published in 1981 and still as valid today as then, described the explosion of litigation and the enormous impact it has on every aspect of American life (no other country has as many lawyers or as many suits or as many problems resulting from them).[5] Yet, we should not try to eliminate or emasculate malpractice. A *reasonable* threat of malpractice suits creates a constructive tension in physicians that helps keep those on the fringe of quality more on their toes.

Furthermore, a well brought and researched malpractice suit can sometimes force changes in entrenched bad practices and methods. Equally important, patients injured by true negligence deserve compensation and justice. Unfortunately, malpractice litigation as it exists today is not reasonable. First, too many malpractice suits are brought for unfortunate results, not for results of negligence. Many obstetricians have stopped delivering babies because they know that if a baby is born with something—anything—wrong, they would be sued even if they had nothing to do with the adverse outcome. In some communities, it is difficult to find a doctor to deliver a child.

Ironically, lawyers miss as many actual occurrences of malpractice as they prosecute contrived ones. Some malpractice goes unrecognized, but other instances are not acted upon because the lawyer feels there is not enough money in it to make it worthwhile. For example, in a suit, "loss" is coldly calculated as years of useful life (based on statistics tables) remaining after the alleged injury and the estimated amount of money the patient could have earned in those years. A very old retired man who is badly injured nevertheless would have a small loss. The suit would be filed only if there was some other factor that could justify a large enough claim to make the suit worthwhile to the lawyer. Actual damages (cost of treatment, lost wages, etc.) are enlarged by penalty multipliers and claims for "anguish and suffering." If a wrongly prescribed medication causes you a temporary severe harm but requires little treatment and no lost work time, you would have too little loss to matter.

Lawyers who defend their right to unlimited suits claim that they are helping society by keeping bad doctors under control. If that were their true purpose, they would allow their clients to sue only negligent doctors and they would sue even if there were a less lucrative award at the end of the rainbow.

I once discussed with a personal injury lawyer the fact that at least ten doctors I know have been sued for malpractice against patients they never knew or ever took care of. In each case, they were sued by mistake. When lawyers sue, to cover every contingency and sometimes to avoid accusations of malpractice on their own part by their clients, they go to excessive lengths, including suing every name on the chart and any others they think might be involved. In some cases, they just sent their subpoenas to the wrong doctor. One doctor I know, a division chief internationally acclaimed in his field, called up and told the lawyer cheerfully that he had mistaken him for a first-year surgery resident whose name was the same as his. He stopped smiling when the lawyer said, "Prove it in court," which took him *two years* to do! Another friend, one of the most senior and distinguished physicians at the medical center, was wrongly named in another suit. It took a total of *ten* hours of pretrial discovery testimony to convince the lawyers that he had never seen nor heard of the patient.

What was the answer to this from the personal injury lawyer? He said it was a small price for one citizen to pay for another to gain redress (his word) for an injured party. Now remember, these are very busy doctors whose lives and practices were seriously disrupted, not to mention the significant emotional stress over cases in which they were totally uninvolved but for the error of the lawyer. I do not think the doctors felt it was a "small" price.

Excessive lawsuits damage society, as Lieberman has well documented, and distort medical practice. Malpractice imposes a severe drain on health care resources.[6] The yearly cost of lawyers, trials, malpractice insurance, and payments for successful claims or settlements runs in the $10–15 billion dollar category, *not* including the cost of the time lost by defendant physicians, and has been increasing by about eight times faster than lawsuits in general. This is magnified manyfold by the cost of defensive medicine, which, while impossible to estimate accurately, probably adds many billions more to the bills we pay each year. "Defensive medicine," which we will discuss shortly, occurs when doctors order additional, unnecessary tests solely to protect against a potential legal action that they cannot anticipate but want to preclude in any way they can.

Though lawsuits against physicians are increasing by as much as 12 percent per year, defendant physicians win *80 percent* of all cases that go to trial. Seventy percent of all claims filed against physicians do *not* result in payment to the plaintiff.

There are assertions that *true* malpractice occurs much more often than what is brought to court and that there are hundreds of thousands of injuries and deaths due to incompetent medical treatment.[7] The truth depends on how "injury," "cause," "fault," and "responsibility" are defined. These studies are done by researchers reviewing patients' medical records and reaching judgments based on their interpretation of what they read. What are the biases of the reviewers? How badly did they want to find fault? What statistical manipulations were used?

While we should do everything in our power to minimize error and negligence, from my experience and interviews I do not believe that there is an army of doctors and nurses damaging people all over the country.

There is an enormous challenge ahead of us. Hospital care is incredibly complex and the problem is multiplied manyfold by the fact that so many people are involved in patient care. We will discuss how to apply modern technology to reduce medication errors and other mistakes, but endless litigation—whose only goal is money or publicity—is not the answer.

On the other end of the spectrum, individual practitioners can get out of touch with their colleagues and the vital information flow, or get sloppy and complacent. That results in bad care as much as the overloading of the system. This likewise must be addressed, but constructively, not destructively for profit. We will discuss this in the last chapter.

Doctors practicing "defensive medicine" must order more tests, do more procedures, and advise patients of ever more lengthy lists of risks in order that a lawyer will not look back years later and criticize some alleged omission. Adverse results occur no matter how good the medical care, but it is possible for a plaintiff's lawyer to present a case in a way that could make any doctor look guilty.

This well-recognized phenomenon exposes patients to unnecessary tests, anxiety, and expense, which managed care is supposed to reduce. Managed care would argue that they improve care and provide oversight that would counteract defensive medicine, but I doubt if they succeed. Their motive, of course, is more likely just to save money, since they seldom have to worry about lawsuits, although that is likely to change soon.

Suppose a patient comes and asks about a lump on her upper back. The doctor examines it and concludes it is a harmless lipoma, which, as we discussed previously, is benign almost every time. As we said, such lesions should be biopsied only if they feel unusual in some way or if they change or grow rapidly.

Suppose that this lump is the even rarer case which is malignant but gives no indication of being so. When the diagnosis is eventually made, the reaction should be unhappiness that such an unusual circumstance occurred. What could occur instead would be a lawsuit in which a lawyer presented the facts in such a way as to convince a jury that a negligent error had occurred. To avoid the possibility of such an error, doctors would have to remove *all* lipomas. Assuming that each American has an average of two, that would mean 520 million surgeries. This extreme extension of the principle illustrates what happens when external interference replaces individual judgment.

Malpractice insurance carriers send an endless stream of advice on avoiding malpractice to physicians they insure. Some of it pertains to good medical practice. Much of it amounts to an endless restatement of the simple concept: How will this look and sound in court?

A relatively new legal threat to doctors is from publicity-hungry local prosecutors. Doctors and nurses are being charged with felonies where once the only legal action would have been a civil action, malpractice. Mark Crane, senior editor of *Medical Economics* magazine, described several of these cases recently; these descriptions are based on his reporting.[8] One doctor, Gerald Einaugler, was actually sent to jail in a highly disputable case that was certainly no criminal act. The case began in 1990 with the care of a seventy-eight-year old woman in a nursing home who developed complications from a treatment. She appeared stable in the morning and he felt she could be safely monitored in the nursing home. As the day progressed, she seemed to worsen and at the end of the day Einaugler arranged her transfer to the hospital. The woman died four days later. He was not accused of causing or contributing to her death and there was no evidence that his actions hastened it. He was indicted and convicted of two misdemeanor counts of reckless endangerment and neglect for not having transferred her *sooner* that day. There is considerable question whether his actions were even bad judgment, but in any case that is what his decision was, an exercise of medical judgment within the bounds of medical discretion. Were there question as to his judgment being negligent, the appropriate forum was civil court, not criminal court. He did nothing criminal and certainly did not deserve the jail time he endured. The case remains under appeal eight years after the event; he has been through a tortuous experience and his career has been destroyed.

In another case, in 1991, a Miami family physician was charged with manslaughter and "abuse of the elderly" after the death of a diabetic. The prosecutor called a press conference and made front-page news. When it was discovered that the doctor was not even in the state when the alleged abuse occurred, the doctor was completely vindicated but it was barely reported. His thirty-year career was ruined. "Who wants a doctor who's been accused of murder?" he said. There are other examples as well in which careers are destroyed by medical judgments being prosecuted as criminal acts, most of which resulted in acquittal or dismissal in favor of the defendants.

There is a continuing theme here. Current remedies intended to help only make the problem worse. There *are* too many errors in medicine and the system *does* need radical improvement, but there are better and worse ways to do it. We will discuss the right way in chapter 14.

Here we have been discussing how the law is being misapplied. Should the insurance companies be above the law? Should a lawyer's desire for one-third of a settlement dictate how your doctor treats you? There must be, and there is, a better way.

NOTES

1. Laurie Zoloth-Dorfman and Susan Rubin, "The Patient as Commodity: Managed Care and the Question of Ethics," *Journal of Clinical Ethics* 6 (Winter 1995): 339–57.

2. Health Care Liability Alliance website, http://www.wp.com/hela, May 10, 1998.

3. David L. Coleman, "Will Health Plans Keep Their ERISA Shield?" *Managed Care* (May 1997), downloaded August 11, 1998, from http://www.managedcaremag.com/archiveMC/9705/9705.erisa.shtml.

4. Ibid.

5. Jethro K. Lieberman, *The Litigious Society* (New York: Basic Books, 1981).

6. Health Care Liability Alliance website, May 10, 1998.

7. Michael L. Millenson, *Demanding Medical Excellence* (Chicago: University of Chicago Press, 1997).

8. Mark Crane, "Medical Convictions," *Reason* 30 (May 1998): 44–48.

11

How Managed Care Bypasses, Controls, and Limits Doctors to Save Money and Why You Pay the Price

Doctors earn high incomes and thus are seen as a drain on health care resources and the profits of managed care companies. Managed care costs could be reduced if the companies could find ways to deliver care with less expensive practitioners. The companies also try to reduce their costs by pushing the doctors in their networks to comply with the way they practice medicine by issuing guidelines that serve as a kind of cookbook. We will examine why that is not good. Managed care companies have bought many hospitals and converted them from nonprofit to profit. We will discuss the implications of this. We will explore why alternative medicine is seen as a cost-cutting opportunity and what problems it entails. We will also explore some problems related to the pharmaceutical industry, Medicare, and Medicaid, as all these impact managed care and the whole health care system with which we are concerned.

To better understand how medical care can be impaired by erosion of physicians' roles, we first need to see what goes into educating and training good doctors.

What does it take to become a doctor? Let us follow a young woman in high school who decides she wants to go to medical school and practice medicine. First, she must score very high on her SAT exams and be at the top of her class in high school to get into a good college. Then she must be at the very top of her class in four years of college and score high on the major achievement exams to get into medical school. Depending on the school and decade, there are from *three to ten applicants for every medical school opening.* Those who cannot get into an American school can attend a foreign school instead, but that path is less prestigious and the education is more limited.

Once accepted in medical school, the student faces a daunting task. There are few pursuits in life as difficult and demanding as medical school and the subsequent hospital training. The competition is extremely high, the physical and intellectual demands are exhausting, and there is enormous emotional strain.

There are two parts to medical school: the didactic (the lectures and exams that teach the science behind medical care) and the clinical experience. The lectures and laboratory work include the following:

- *Anatomy* studies the parts of the body. Crucial to the study is the six-month-long dissection of an actual human body. Thus, in the first year, the student, who came from college, football games, dates, and the like, is confronted by death and the necessary invasion of the intimate privacy of another person's body.
- *Histology* studies what normal human tissue looks like under the microscope.
- *Pathology* studies what abnormal organs and tissue look like.
- *Organic chemistry* studies the chemistry of life.
- *Physiology* studies how the chemical processes in the body work together to make life.
- *Pharmacology* studies how medications and other substances work and how they interact with each other and with the chemistry of the body.
- *Microbiology* studies how bacteria, viruses, and fungi cause disease and how they can be studied, fought, and prevented.
- *Physical diagnosis* teaches the skills of examining a patient (often practicing on other students) and history taking.
- Other courses concentrate on individual subjects such as *public health, preventive medicine, nutrition,* and medical specialties.
- Many schools today give special courses on *ethics, how to communicate* with patients, and other essentials of good medical care.

Each of these courses is taught at the same level as for doctoral (Ph.D.) candidates and requires learning and memorizing enormous amounts of facts, names, and concepts, all tested on huge exams.

Then there is the clinical experience, which derives from William Osler's dictum, mentioned before, to take the student to the bedside. It used to be that the first two years of medical school were lectures and laboratory work and the last two comprised clinical work, but many schools today begin clinical experience in the first year interspersed with the didactic courses.

In clinical training, students wear short white coats and work on the wards of the hospitals and in the outpatient clinics. There they begin to see patients under close supervision of a senior doctor. The supervisor may be a postgraduate trainee or an attending physician ("attending" means a doctor who has finished all training and is accredited to be on the hospital staff).

The adjustment from college student to caregiver, holding the lives of people in one's hands, in an incubator of extremely high activity, pressure, and stress, is startling. There is competition among students that forces them to at least look as if they know it all.

There is the pressure of the house staff, who have just come through it and figure, "If *I* did it, I'm going to make you prove *you* are up to it." There are cultural differences among hospitals and medical centers, but many schools have a macho, prove-you-can-make-it atmosphere. It is not unlike marine boot camp, only there are live microbes instead of live ammunition. The idea is that if our student can survive, she is tough enough to make it in medicine. (Medicine was long a male-dominated society and, to its shame, women were subjected to pressures and treatment their male counterparts did not suffer. Women are now a significant percentage of the student body and, I hope, modern concepts of equality have reached the schools and hospitals.)

There is a significant dropout rate in medical school, both voluntary and requested, but if our student survives and graduates, she has a coveted M.D. degree. She then begins postgraduate training. What used to be called internship is now less elegantly referred to as PGY-1 (postgraduate year 1; residency is now PGY-2, and so on).

In internship (I personally will stick to the old terms), the student is a full-time hospital employee responsible for the care of a group of patients. She is closely supervised by residents (more senior housestaff trainees), attending doctors who teach housestaff, and the patients' private doctors, who have the primary authority for the care of their own patients.

The intern admits patients to the hospital, which means she evaluates them, takes a complete history and physical exam, orders initial tests and treatments, and advises the patient about what is happening. She then follows her patients' orders, tests, and treatments; talks to the patients and to the attending doctors and consultants; and does the busy work connected to patient care: drawing blood for tests, starting intravenous lines, getting lab results, obtaining specimens, and all the other small but critical parts of patient care.

All this takes an enormous amount of time and energy, while at the same time the interns and residents have to deal successfully with the senior doctors, nurses, aides, technicians, and the patients' families. They attend teaching "rounds" where a group circulates among all the patients, each intern presenting a summary of the individual patient's progress and answering questions about the patient or relevant medical facts. The housestaff have to be prepared to answer any and all questions not only about the patient's condition, but about the science background and the latest findings in the medical literature.

Illness does not follow nine-to-five hours. Medicine is a twenty-four-hour day. Housestaff officers are on duty alternating nights and usually get little or no sleep when they are on duty. Following patients through *every* aspect of their care is a vital part of learning. You simply have no time or interest in anything except what is happening on your ward. You may be on duty for thirty-six hours nonstop.

When I was doing hospital work, we learned how to do procedures by the rule of "watch one, do one, teach one." This applied to *everything*: liver biopsies, drawing fluid out of lungs, spinal taps, and the like. This kind of practical experience is much harder to come by in today's litigious climate.

Most patients today would not knowingly let a student learn on them. In practice, the process actually worked and I saw few if any adverse consequences of student care. We can never go back to the old way and there are now only a few hospitals where the housestaff continue to have such primary care of the patients. The question arises, however, whether we are training doctors as well as we did when they had the chance to have more hands-on experience.

A major issue today is how we train young doctors while at the same time preserving the patients' rights to the best care. Part of the answer is that properly supervised students and housestaff give excellent care and often contribute in very positive ways to the patient's benefit.

The key is the supervision. One of the many prices we pay for managed care and Medicare is the damage to medical education. Hospital reimbursements have been severely restricted by managed care and Medicare, which has reduced funds for education and research. Doctors have less time to supervise students and housestaff, as they must work harder to maintain income. Medical schools may not retain faculty as the hospital's financial condition deteriorates. As doctors are driven from academic medicine and the time of those remaining becomes so limited, who will train the doctors of the future?

The demands of medical training are great and sleep is a luxury. New York State passed a law limiting the number of hours that housestaff can work because of an infamous case where a fatal mistake was allegedly made partly due to housestaff sleep deprivation. The compliance rate with this law is low.

Pushing housestaff to such extremes of exhaustion that they make life-threatening mistakes is obviously not acceptable, but every effort should be made not to damage the alchemy of turning a raw student into a seasoned caregiver.

Physicians do not climb the nearly impossible mountain of becoming a doctor driven by desire for money or power. Only a meaningful calling can sustain someone through such a challenge. I spent eight years in medical school, internship, residency, and fellowship studies. No one told me to work hard or to do anything. They did not need to. The other students and I drove ourselves harder than anyone else possibly could. When you realize that you hold other people's lives in your hands, the responsibility is so overwhelming that you never stop giving everything you have to be the very best you can be.

Well, our student has now graduated medical school and holds a Doctor of Medicine degree, but she cannot practice medicine except as an intern in the hospital. To be licensed, she must successfully pass one or two years of postgraduate training, depending on the state, and pass a licensing exam.

Once licensed, she can practice medicine, but if she wants to be recognized as a specialist, she must undertake additional training as a resident doctor in the hospital. That can take from two more years to as much as seven more years in some surgical subspecialties. To be a subspecialist requires several to many post-internship years as a resident and fellow. To specialize in internal medicine requires three postgraduate years and another two years of what is called a fellowship to be a subspecialist in heart disease, infectious disease, etc. Neurosurgery can take as much as seven to nine postgraduate years. Specialties include internal medicine, pediatrics, obstetrics and gynecology, and family practice. These four are commonly called primary care, since the doctor that most patients think of as their main doctor is usually from one of these specialties.

Family practice is a relatively new specialty in which practitioners are trained to do what the old general practitioners used to do—medicine, pediatrics, minor surgery, some obstetrics, and orthopedics, except that unlike the old way, they do a residency with abbreviated periods of training in each of those fields.

There are of course many other specialties, including all the surgical fields, radiology, pathology, anesthesiology, dermatology, neurology, and more. All of the specialties now have major exams, which take two or more full days, and sets of qualifications, which, if successfully completed and passed, allow one to be certified as a specialist. This is called being board certified or a diplomate. As an example, I am a diplomate of the American Board of Internal Medicine.

Being certified does not guarantee one is a good doctor. It does certify that one is a good exam taker, but the exams cannot really reproduce clinical situations, try as they might, and therefore do not fully reflect clinical skills. They also do not measure the quality of the examinee's character. Having said all that, board certification is still a worthwhile credential to look for in a doctor, though it ignores some fine physicians who may fail the exams or just not take them but whose years of experience have taught more than can be measured by an exam.

Once our student finishes her training and passes all her exams, she begins the next phase of her study, which is the rest of her life. Medicine is too much to learn even in the long formal education and training period. You never learn everything and you learn new and anew every day. In addition, the rate of change and growth in medical knowledge is so rapid that she must keep up with the continual changes on a daily basis.

* * *

Now, having understood all that goes into learning medicine, how would you like instead to go to someone who has had a fraction of this training and education?

Suppose you have a cold. Why not go to someone less expensive? You might see a nurse practitioner or a physician's assistant. They have had some college and two to three years of training in their field. My concern is whether they will give as good care as a physician.

For example, I saw a thirty-six-year-old father of six, a middle management executive, in a clinic. He complained of a cold. He felt a little weak, had some sniffles, a sore throat, a little cough, and a low-grade fever. I examined him, then took the next hour to convince him to go to the hospital. He was reluctant to go to so much trouble for what seemed like a little cold, as most people would be.

When I examined him, I had heard a moderately loud heart

murmur and the previous clinic notes had described a murmur that was less intense. A normal heart beat sounds something like *lub–dub.* A murmur may sound like *lub–ssshhh–dub.* That shushing sound may indicate an abnormality in one of the four valves in the heart. Ordinarily, the volume of the sound is not necessarily meaningful, but in the presence of an infection, an increase in the volume of the sound may indicate that the infection has settled on the lip of the damaged valve, though sometimes fever alone makes it seem louder. However, an infection in the heart, called endocarditis, is so serious that it must be checked out. Treated early, complete recovery is possible, but delay can bring severe damage, surgery to replace the valve, or even death.

In the hospital, it was confirmed that he had endocarditis caused by an uncommon organism, but after extended treatment, he recovered fully. Had I originally just sent him home with a few nostrums for his cold symptoms, the endocarditis might have progressed beyond the point of a good result. Had he mistakenly been given antibiotics, the infection would have been masked but not cured (endocarditis requires a long course of intravenous, high-dose antibiotics) and he would have eventually done very poorly.

I have picked up other such cases as well, also very early, with excellent results. Would a lesser trained practitioner have done so? What seems like a common cold can be many different serious, even life-threatening illnesses. Only a small percentage are, but that is where the skill and care count—to find the important few among the many, to be alert for small signs, to be so careful that you do not miss the needle in the haystack.

Countless times patients have come for minor complaints and I have been able to redirect their attention to serious problems. It may be a deadly skin cancer on the knee that is removed in the nick of time. A doctor may detect subtle signs of diabetes the patient did not know he had. A little blood in the stool that the patient thinks is just hemorrhoids could be an intestinal growth called a polyp, perhaps with an early cancer. Convincing a patient to go for a colonoscopy, inserting a fiberoptic tube into the bowel, allows removal of a polyp with a cancer so early it is curable by the office procedure alone.

A lesser trained practitioner may be dedicated and brilliant, but he or she cannot learn in abbreviated training what is forged in the crucible of the full medical training described previously.

Why such a long and impassioned discussion of this topic? It is that these alternative practitioners are *cheaper* to hire than doctors and are therefore the apple of every HMO's eye. If cold accounting is all that matters, doctors appear to be an unnecessary expense. Just hire these other folks, give them little cookbooks called clinical guidelines, and that's all you need. Keep a few specialists on hand for show, and, of course for when the HMO executives themselves get sick, but otherwise replace them all! That may seem like a sarcastic exaggeration, but there actually have been many serious proposals to solve health care costs by replacing doctors with alternative practitioners and using doctors only for the most severe problems. Recall in chapter 2 Victor Fuch's idea to divide care of patients between doctors as curers and less expensive personnel as carers. A New York City hospital is currently sponsoring a group of nurse practitioners who practice independently of doctors at lower fees. Bills are regularly introduced in the New York State legislature attempting to extend physician functions to other professions such as optometrists, chiropractors, physician assistants, and nurse practitioners

One of the television newsmagazines did a show on a nonprofit HMO. Its reporter interviewed the executive who ran the company. He was very angry about "expensive" doctors. He said neurosurgeons had some nerve charging so much money. He bragged about how many doctors he had replaced with assistants, nurse practitioners, and even lesser-trained aides and said he was working toward eliminating doctors from the system *completely*.

At the end of the piece, the reporter quietly noted that this *nonprofit* executive was making three times as much money as the neurosurgeons on his staff. Keep in mind that neurosurgery requires up to *nine* years of postgraduate training, that one surgery can take ten to fifteen hours, and that there is *no* room for error, a stressful job matched by little else. The executive, depicted in a TV report, does not represent all managed care and may be since long gone, but the temptation to look for cheaper alternatives exists and efforts to find substitutes will undoubtedly continue.

Nurse practitioners and physician assistants are lobbying hard for the right to practice independently of doctors, to prescribe medications, and to admit patients to the hospital. In New York State, they already have some of these rights. If they succeed in replacing doctors, will they find

- the meningitis case among the hundreds of headaches?
- the endocarditis among the endless colds?
- the patient with a stiff neck who is at risk of paralysis among the many who just need simple care?

- the small lymph node that allows early detection of a cancer?
- the subtle variation in texture that hides a breast cancer?
- the seemingly innocent stomachache that is an appendix about to rupture?
- the little pain in the grandfather's side that is really a serious intestinal infection?

The following table contains a sample selection of how difficult even the simplest seeming cases can be:

A patient who comes to a doctor thinking he or she has just a cold could actually have many different possible conditions. Here is just a partial list:

1. Viral infections, such as common cold, measles, rubella
2. Bacterial infections
3. Rocky Mountain Spotted Fever
4. Lyme Disease
5. Pneumonia
6. Asthma
7. Hay fever
8. Postnasal drip causing cough
9. Sinusitis
10. Congestive heart failure
11. Endocarditis
12. Meningitis
13. Dehydration syndrome
14. Heart attack
15. Pulmonary embolus (blood clot to lung)

All of these could progress to serious, even life-threatening complications. Some can be fatal within minutes or hours.

No visit is truly simple, all patients are important, and every patient deserves the highest level of care.

Only medical school and hospital training provide the experience and the foundation that comprise good medical care. They are not perfect—what is?—but they are the best preparation for the care of patients we have available.

One doctor I interviewed was trying to help a friend who finished a pediatric residency at a major medical center. Managed care has so changed medical economics that some physicians are having great difficulty finding positions. He could not find a reasonable job. The few possibilities available had salaries around $60,000, which is the range for physician assistants after a few years of experience. Do we really want to lower our standards and undervalue physicians? Sixty thousand dollars is a lot of money to many people and should be treated with respect, but for the investment in time, the debts incurred, the skill required, the risk undertaken, physicians' services should be valued appropriately. In the next chapter we discuss the difficult question of what value to put on physicians' services.

Nonphysician practitioners are a valuable addition to the medical team when they work closely with physicians on specifically designated tasks. They are vital in rural areas where there are few physicians. They provide invaluable home care services in outreach programs. They have important roles in doctors' offices and other areas. As highly as I regard these practitioners, they are not physicians and they should not be used as substitutes just to save money. I am sure that these words will elicit much protest from many fine practitioners, but I think patients will have to judge for themselves what kind of training they want for *their* care.

PRACTICE GUIDELINES

We are becoming a digital world. More and more information and processes are rapidly being converted to bits of information. What most people are unaware of is that all digital information is based on yes/no paths known as algorithms.

"Algorithm" has come into common use to mean a type of simplified guideline to describe a process and some of the choices and alternatives available. It begins with a path and offers branching choices. If yes, you proceed one way, if no, then you head in another. Each stage is a yes/no or equivalent decision. Do you want potatoes with your dinner? If yes, do you want a baked potato? If no, do you want French fried potatoes? If yes, do you want ketchup with them?

You do not live your life algorithmically. Your brain most likely works partly in a digital yes/no method, but your thinking processes are undoubtedly far more complex. How we think, learn, and create involves far more than simple algorithms. The more connections between the nerve cells of our brain, the better we can think. Albert Einstein's brain was normal in size and weight. Scientists for a long time could not detect a difference that explained his brilliance (he had willed his brain to science for study). Not long ago, they were finally able to analyze the number of nerve connections. Einstein's brain had significantly larger numbers of complex connections than the average human. This larger number of pathways may indicate that Einstein accessed information in a variety of ways, allowing him to recombine data and thereby make the postulations and discoveries for which he is famous. His brain lends weight to the theory that there are very likely aspects of thought that are not digital, not just yes/no. Intuition, imagination, love, and a sense of beauty likely transcend what we currently understand from computer logic.

Certain skills can be learned in a digital, structured way: assembling machinery, washing dishes, simple arithmetic, filing documents. Other skills must be learned on a higher level by experience. Each person will do so in his or her own, unique way. Examples include playing baseball, heart surgery, higher mathematics, playing the violin, teaching. A third type of skill cannot be learned, only developed: creativity, such as what differentiates ordinary and good painting, poetry, music—and the care of patients.

As we study for our occupations, each of us develops in his or her own way. We each bring our own history, experience, beliefs, previous knowledge, emotions, and goals into our choice of profession. I mention this because a cookbook mentality cannot work in medicine. Even cookbooks for cooks are just a starting point. Few people would enjoy a meal I made from a recipe book because I have no cooking skills; my wife, however, can make a sumptuous meal from the same book.

There is a large body of literature describing the variations in treatment among doctors, hospitals, and regions of the country. One city will have twice the rate of hysterectomies as another or one hospital will treat most angina with surgery while another uses medical treatment far more often. Michael Millenson discusses these problems at some length in his book *Demanding Medical Excellence*,[1] in which he discusses problems he feels medicine has inadequately addressed.

Which is right? The operators or the prescribers? Part of the problem is the studies themselves. There are differences in the mixes of patients and in other factors that may influence the differences in treatment. Certainly some of the differences are due simply to differences in point of view.

Critics of medicine assume that if one hospital does more surgery, the only reason it could be is that that hospital wants to make more money, just as it appears that managed care reduces procedures to save themselves money.

There is some truth in this, as unnecessary surgery does occur. One case I know of is illustrative. A seventy-five-year-old woman was dying of uterine cancer. She had weeks to live and was in great pain. An intern noted a skin lesion on her back. It was diagnosed as an advanced malignant melanoma. A highly respected surgeon insisted on removing it. The skin cancer was not bothering her and was not a risk that would bother her for possibly years later, but she was close to death from the uterine cancer. The operation caused her more unnecessary discomfort and cost $900.

Did the surgeon do it for the money, or was he just thoughtless? Either reason was wrong.

I believe, based on my experience, that the degree of excessive procedures just to make money, while needing attention, has been exaggerated. Far more often, the surgeons and other procedural doctors I have worked with over the years have been very conservative in treating patients. They do not operate or perform a procedure unless the patient absolutely needs it and there is no better option. I never order anything for which I do not have a specific, imperative reason. For each doctor who operates selfishly or unnecessarily, I believe there are many more who do not.

Another major problem is keeping doctors up to date and their skills honed. Equally important is to ensure that all doctors practice in a sound and good way. I have supervised many doctors, including medical students, housestaff, staff doctors, and doctors who have gotten in trouble.*

Doctors are among the hardest people to supervise. The very qualities that make good doctors make them resistant to easy supervision. Most doctors are the last of the rugged individualists. They are not followers. They question everything, do not operate by assumptions and are continuously questioning and rethinking. Doctors also realize that they must achieve their ability to care for patients by synthesizing a broad array of factors, such as what they learn in school, what they read daily, what teachers and colleagues contribute, and what their own experience has taught. Included in the mix are their own beliefs and backgrounds and all that they learn from every patient.

In my experience, doctors do not simply begin to do what you teach them. What goes in comes out in each doctor's unique inte-

---

*New York State agencies that discipline doctors call on experienced physicians to help them improve their practices. In addition, a doctor may observe that a colleague needs help in some areas.

grated formulation. Nonphysicians observe the medical world and see what looks to them like organized chaos. They want to bring order, regularity and conformity. They try to impose their own idea of order. It does not work.

Managed care and Medicare have forced medicine into a new field—clinical guidelines. These are cookbook-like descriptions of how to take care of medical conditions, whether a urinary tract infection or a stroke. Sometimes the descriptions are in outline form and sometimes they are algorithm charts with little boxes, yeses and nos and lots of lines.

That is not how to change medicine. Taking care of people is a practice not susceptible to management techniques designed for assembly lines and financial interactions. There are simply too many uncontrollable variables. It is like a two-armed man trying to wrestle an eight-armed octopus—the octopus is six arms ahead, and, in its own environment, much smarter. Guidelines are one small piece of educational literature, which, if used only that way, are fine. Unfortunately, like everything else in managed care, they are becoming tools of control and cost containment.

Guidelines are written by committees. The old joke is that a zebra is a horse designed by a committee. That is not quite accurate. A committee would create a creature that was half horse and half zebra, since the members would be divided fifty-fifty and would settle it with a compromise. The thing would have a backside at both ends and it would not know if it was coming or going.

There is truth in the world, but we can never discover *the* truth. We discover what we see as truth, while others may see it entirely differently. A committee has to resolve these differences, which it does by compromise. It arrives at a report that half-pleases everyone but completely pleases no one. Truth is not achieved by majority vote. Compromises settle disputes but have nothing to do with finding truth.

If an individual produces something, that is truth as he or she sees it and the product has integrity. The individual then presents it to the group, which criticizes and suggests, but if the individual retains control, even if agreeing with many of the suggestions, the result may retain integrity. Compromises have no integrity, only peacefulness.

This may all sound highly theoretical and philosophical and may seem to have nothing to do with affordable health care, but it has vitally real consequences. Once an agency has created a guideline, it becomes a requirement. Deviations are punished. A cardiologist colleague of mine says that today, if a patient arrives in the emergency room with a stroke, that patient must receive every step on the protocol even if a given procedure is unnecessary or wrong for that particular case. Later review may indicate that there was deviation from the guideline and the transgressor would be punished. It will not matter that there may have been excellent reasons why the guidelines were not applicable in that case and that the situation may have called for a different approach.

No guideline can cover all contingencies or apply to all patients. Nevertheless, deviation from a guideline may lay the staff open to censure or even a malpractice suit.

Treating patients is a fluid endeavor. The components of each situation change and shift as diagnosis proceeds. No two cardiac arrests are the same, no two asthma attacks are the same, not even colds are the same each time. Physicians and nurses must adjust what they are doing from minute to minute in everything they do, and not just during emergencies.

Guidelines stifle creativity, even though as teaching tools they have some small value. As requirements, they serve only as instruments of control and inhibition of high quality. By issuing a guideline for stroke, for example, the HMO may require more tests than needed, but that cost is more than offset by the shortened length of stay that is the main purpose of the guideline.

Patients in HMOs end up in nursing homes more often, a sign of poor rehabilitation, because they have been discharged from the hospital too early and have been deprived of physical and other therapy that would help them return to a functioning independent life.

The HMOs save money, but the patient and society pay for it by having unnecessarily increased numbers of disabled and dysfunctional people.

HMOs send their doctors endless streams of educational materials. It makes them look good, as if they are promoting quality. In truth, they may talk about promoting a high level of care, but they do not *fund* that level of care. Yet, HMOs hold the doctor accountable for what they *said* to do, not what they *paid* to do.

Such guidelines can be used to save money in other subtle ways. There may be two ways of doing something, but only the less expensive way may appear in the guideline. For example, of two medications for hypertension the more expensive one may be better but the cheaper one is recommended. I do not believe that guidelines promote good care; their disadvantages invalidate their use. The publication may look impressive, but looks can be deceiving.

MEDICAL MARKETING AND THE EROSION OF COLLEGIALITY

Cooperation and lack of financial competitiveness have always been a part of medicine. That is now eroding under managed care. (The rise of biotechnology companies has raised the stakes and the potential for high returns is creating strain in the research world.) One of the concepts behind managed care is that it will increase competition and thus reduce prices. Competition already exists, but other than among HMOs, it is not based on price. Doctors and hospitals are advertising as never before. The art of advertising is to convince and to paint the product in the best light. Advertising is supposed to inform, but who among us trusts what we hear in advertising? What does this do to medicine, where truth and honesty are the hallmarks of quality and ethical practice? Must we sell our birthright to sell our services?

Most managed care ads I have seen paint pictures that are exactly the opposite of what the HMO actually delivers.

When the physician knows that the HMO does not live up to its advertising, is the doctor obligated to inform the patient? What happens if his contract has a gag clause? How does the doctor resolve the conflict between personal financial motive and ethical obligation if huge advertising budgets are at stake?

Cooperation and sharing ideas and knowledge are essential to good medical practice. What happens to that when physicians actively compete for patients and the favors of the HMOs? When referring to a specialist comes out of the referral physician's pocket, how many referrals are made? How do the specialists attract referrals? These kinds of competitive issues are normal for business, but this way of thinking is not appropriate for the delivery of medical care. Dr. Samuel Packer, chairman of the Department of Ophthalmology at North Shore University Hospital, in a paper presented at a symposium on managed care, quotes a business publication: "The decision-making process at top-management levels has little room for social responsibilities not definitely required by law or public opinion."[2] Medicine in contrast should not be a competition for dollars, because social responsibility *is* its first priority.

If you need medical care, you want your doctors to be working together closely and for only one reason: *your* best interests.

JUST WHAT THE DOCTOR ORDERED?

Another HMO approach is "therapeutic substitution." This means that a drug is dispensed that is different than what the doctor prescribed, but supposedly equivalent.

A medical assistant, who was taking an antihypertensive drug called Vasotec, showed me the bottle she received from the pharmacy when she filled a new prescription. It contained Zestril. They are two different drugs, though they are both in a class of drugs known for short as ACE inhibitors. They are similar, but they are not the same. The pharmacist had made the change without even telling her because that was required by her HMO drug plan, as he explained to her when she later questioned him.

First, we have to understand drug terminology: A drug has a chemical name. Let us take an example: 7-(D-a-Amino-a-phenylacetamido)-3-methyl-3-cephem-4-carboxylic acid monohydrate. That does not exactly trip off the tongue. It is given a "generic" name that is a little easier, but still not very salable: cephalexin. It is a member of a class of related drugs, a type of antibiotic called cephalosporins. To make the drug more marketable, the drug company uses computers, focus groups, and naming experts and comes up with a name that is easy to remember: Keflex, a commonly used antibiotic.

A drug can be sold under many different brand names if the original owner licenses it to other companies or if the patent on the formula expires. For example, albuterol inhaler for asthma is sold as Ventolin by one company, Proventil by another, and albuterol as the generic. They are identical in every way except minor differences in the packaging. (The drug salesman for one tried to convince me that I should prescribe his brand because the cap had a small lip that made it easier to grasp. The poor fellow was struggling to find *something* to differentiate his product.)

Next, we have to understand the pharmaceutical industry, one of the highest profit businesses in the country, even though it costs as much as $200 million to bring one new drug to market. Research and development absorb huge sums, and yet many drug candidates do not pan out. The Food and Drug Administration (FDA) requires an extremely extensive testing process to prove that the drug is effective and safe, certainly a function users would endorse wholeheartedly. There are also enormous marketing and distribution costs.

The financial risk of bringing out a new drug is huge because problems—a side effect or other problem not recognized initially—can develop anywhere along the way. There is more risk *after* a new drug passes all the FDA requirements, comes to market, and then gets widely used. Many drugs that seemed harmless in the premarket testing turn out to have some serious risk factor. They may cause kidney or liver damage or problems that are even more serious. Sometimes the effect is bizarre—one drug caused fingernails to peel back and come off. It was quickly withdrawn. There is seldom an explanation as to why the defects do not show up in the preapproval process.

The risks are significant but they pay high rewards. A single drug can earn over $1 billion per year, much of which is profit. The patent rights to exclusive sale extend seventeen years, though some of that is exhausted in the years leading up to approval.

While under patent, the companies spend fortunes marketing the drugs to a tiny audience—the doctors in practice in specialties that use the particular drug. In the past, the marketing amounted to a form of near bribery for some doctors. Expensive trips to conferences at resorts and other kinds of perks were not uncommon. Today, there are limits to this largesse. Most of the giveaways are pens and pads. The drug ads get ever more elaborate. Educational materials are still welcome, including textbooks, models for educating patients, and the like. Honorariums for medical equipment or books of about $100 in value are given for attending meetings or telephone conferences and are not unreasonable compensation for the time spent. I would much prefer that the marketing budgets be reallocated so as to reduce the cost of the drugs, but that will not happen. The marketing works very well. "Detailing," as the sales representative activities are termed, strongly influences many doctors.

Many new drugs are just copycat alternatives to others in the same class, and, without marketing, they would not be profitable. Even the unique and useful drugs get a big boost from marketing. A new approach is to market directly to consumers as well. Although the drugs require a doctor's prescription, the companies hope that patients will see their ads for asthma medications, allergy drugs, or what have you on television and in magazines and then ask their doctors for the medications. It seems to be working and this type of marketing is proliferating.

Another new tactic is that the huge drug store chains now routinely sell *your* private medication information so advertisers and even telemarketers can try to sell you competing or associated brands. Who gave them permission to reveal your private information? If there is no law to cover this unanticipated new approach, there should be.

Pharmaceutical companies are increasingly funding medical schools and medical school research. This is another consequence of managed care. The severe restriction of hospital income has affected the whole medical center, and medical schools are entering into actual partnerships with corporations to undertake research. There is real cause for concern as to what influence the increasing dependence on corporate financing will have on the schools and on research and education.

Once the patent expires on a drug, any company can make it and sell it for lower cost. The mark-up is incredible on brand name drugs. As far back as 1964, Senator Estes Kefauver of Tennessee held congressional hearings on the drug industry and the cost of drugs. Tetracycline, one of the early antibiotics, had been on the market for many years. Testimony revealed that the manufacturer had recouped the costs of development many years before. It cost the company a few mills (a mill is one-thousandth of a cent) to make each pill, yet they charged 75 cents per pill ($3.75 in 1997 dollars). Senator Kefauver expressed great outrage and attempted major reforms, but little actually changed.

Mark-ups continue to be very high. Viagra, a new pill to treat impotence, sells for $10 or more *per pill.* Some new advanced treatments cost hundreds to thousands of dollars per *dose.* These include some hormonal, immune system, and transplant drugs. Drugs for uncommon diseases also cost much more since the volume produced is so much smaller. Some diseases are so rare that no company can afford the investment to develop the drugs for them, but Congress has eased this problem with the passage of the Orphan Drug Act that supports development of high cost–low profit drugs for rare diseases.

A high profit is necessary to stimulate companies to risk so much. Two hundred million dollars is a major risk. The companies claim that any limitation to high return for risk will stifle innovation. However, a number of valuable drugs are developed in Europe and elsewhere and adopted by American companies in joint licensing agreements that spare the licensee the massive cost of development and approval. Furthermore, many drug company developments begin in government-financed university research, independent labs that receive government funding, and the government's own research facilities such as the National Institutes of Health. There has been some discussion that the government should get some share of the profits in return for this virtual subsidy.

There are far fewer controls on drug clearance in other countries. The FDA halted the entry of thalidomide into the United States in the early 1960s because of the high occurrence of birth defects that resulted from its use. The specter of a similar drug getting past the controls and entering wide usage still haunts the FDA decades later. (Thalidomide is being reintroduced as an anti-inflammatory drug for certain conditions but with rigid precautions to prevent it being used in pregnant women.)

Barriers to drug approval have been eased somewhat, but remain very tight. Critics claim that more people suffer from the delay in access to valuable new drugs than might experience adverse effects from a drug cleared too easily. The FDA is trying to satisfy both needs —safety and rapid access—by improving the assessment process. There has been a major increase in speed to market and an unprecedented flood of new drugs. So far, no major disasters have occurred, but there has been an upswing in drugs being withdrawn from use due to adverse effects, even deaths, from problems not recognized before they began to be used widely. Sixteen drugs have been withdrawn from the market since 1980, but four additional ones were pulled just during the past year. Duract, a painkiller, withdrawn June 1998, has been linked to eight liver transplants and four deaths. Posicor, used to treat high blood pressure, has potentially life-threatening interactions with at least twenty-six other drugs and was withdrawn in the same month. Seldane, an antihistamine, was withdrawn in March 1998 after reports of rare but life-threatening drug interactions when taken with other common drugs, such as the widely used antibiotic, erythromycin. Fenfluramine and dexenfluramine, used in the combination known as Fen-fen as an appetite suppressant, turned out to cause serious heart valve damage in as much as one-third of people taking it.[3]

The price of drugs remains a major burden on many people of limited means. For example, a single ten-day course of some brand name antibiotics can cost $90 to $150. The lives of older people especially are often dependent on a large number of drugs. How does someone living on Social Security afford hundreds of dollars of medication costs per month? Medicare does *not* pay for medications. Many of the elderly poor are on Medicaid, which pays for medications, but many others definitely *are* in a bind, especially those who just miss qualifying for Medicaid.

Some HMOs enticed Medicare patients into managed care with the promise of prescription drug programs that would make medications much more affordable. Some of these companies have canceled or cut back on these drug plans after signing up enrollees based on their promise.

Some drug company policies seem impossible to justify. A very old drug that was used widely in agriculture as a food additive for animals sold for $6 per pound. After years of research in university labs, without a penny of pharmaceutical money, it was found to be a helpful adjunct to a particular cancer therapy. It sold as a medication for $6 *per pill.*

Another example is an old cancer drug that was found by university researchers to be a good anti-inflammatory agent for rheumatoid arthritis, psoriasis, and some other diseases. In addition, it only has to be taken in small doses once per week. When used in higher doses for cancer, it is given in much longer courses. The drug now costs more for the small dose once per week regimen than it did for the cancer treatment.

Drug companies justify these practices by the risk they face and the pressures from the investors and stock analysts to maintain their historically high dividends. As I said, I believe we need strong incentives to stimulate research, but I would urge pharmaceutical companies to exercise some restraint for the benefit of those whose need for care is being compromised by very high prices.

A challenge for managed care is to reduce medication costs because the pharmaceutical industry is formidably powerful. Surely, there must be some middle ground among price controls, to which I object strenuously, the need to stimulate research and development, the principle of capitalism, and the contrast of drug prices so high that they exact too great a toll on too many people. Pharmaceutical companies say that they charge what the market will bear, but having a monopoly on a product on which customers' very lives depend is not a *free* market.

Large corporations have been formed to process drug orders by mail. The American Association of Retired Persons (AARP) has a giant mail order operation for its huge membership. However, drug companies have taken over some processors and have used their ownership to influence sales of their own brands.[4]

Managed care and huge hospital corporations have used their economic power to win discounts from drug companies on some products. It is like a battle of behemoths.

Once a drug loses its patent protection, any other manufacturer can then produce and sell it. These are called generic drugs. The secondary producer has none of the development costs and little marketing, since the drugs are marketed directly to pharmacies. The prices are as low as 10 percent of the cost of the brand drug.

Generic substitution has been a long-standing process in most states. In New York, with which I am most familiar, a pharmacist is required by law to dispense a generic form of a drug, if it exists, unless the doctor specifies, "DAW," which means "dispense as written." If a doctor prescribes Keflex, the pharmacist will dispense a generic cephalexin. Doctors know this and can specify the brand if there is a reason to do so.

In many cases, the generic drug is equivalent to the brand drug. In some cases, the same company that sells the brand version manufactures the pills for the generic sellers. Independent producers make others. In those cases, the binders and coatings may be different.

One issue is bioavailability. What matters is how much drug is absorbed into the system and that may vary among different forms of the same drug. For some drugs, such as digitalis, a heart drug, the therapeutic window is very small. That means that the difference between a safe and effective dose is very close to levels that are toxic. Bioavailability is critical with this kind of drug and it is important to adjust the level and maintain it with the exact same drug. The brand name drug has a real advantage in this case.

As a practitioner, it is a great relief to me when some drugs become available generically, because it makes them much more affordable for patients with limited means. On the other hand, I have no way of knowing which company will make the generic, nor its reliability. New York State evaluates all generic drugs and clears them for use.

Like everything else in health care, the story is not quite so simple. What could be better or cheaper than generics? Well, for one thing, newer drugs, still under brand protection, are often easier to take, more effective, safer, and less likely to have side effects. Ease of use is very important because the compliance rate of drug use is abysmally low. Most people find it very difficult to take medications regularly and on schedule. It is obviously much harder to keep to a four-times-a-day regimen than a once-a-day schedule.

When patients fail to take their drugs correctly, the drugs often do not work, causing either a treatment failure or a relapse, sometimes allowing major, unnecessary complications to occur. That may end up much more expensive than the higher cost of the easier-to-comply-with brand would have been.

Another example is a type of calcium channel blocker. These are useful drugs for hypertension and angina, as well as some other conditions. The original drug is available as an inexpensive generic, but it has to be taken three to four times a day. Even more important, serious questions have arisen about its safety. Those concerns remain controversial at this point, but the new, long-acting forms of the drug are not only easier to take, they seem much less likely to have the risks that may apply to the short-acting form. Thus, generics may be valuable in some cases but penny-wise, pound-foolish at other times.

HMOs make no such fine distinctions. Drug plans that dispense medications for a modest copayment increase the availability of drugs, but, like everything else with managed care, the drugs may come at a price that could exceed their value. Slavishly using only generics wherever possible, denying needed drugs that are more expensive because they treat rarer diseases, substituting drugs without permission, or pestering a doctor to use a different drug just to save money—all have significant adverse effects.

There are many examples, but we will examine only one. Tagamet was the first drug that reduced acid production in the stomach. It healed ulcers faster and better than anything previously available and relieved heartburn for many patients. It was soon found, however, that older patients did not tolerate the drug as well. Some would become sleepy or have nightmares or other forms of impaired cognition. That limited Tagamet's use for a major segment of patients. Then it was discovered that Tagamet affected certain enzymes in the liver, causing problems with other drugs, what are called adverse drug interactions.

Then researchers found that if they removed a small portion of the molecule that contained what is called a sulfhydryl group, a chemical component well known to cause problems, the drug worked even better, was easier to take, did not have the adverse effects on older patients and had few, if any, drug interactions. It is sold as Zantac.

Tagamet is still a good drug when precautions are taken against the above problems, and the pharmaceutical company has reduced the price of Tagamet considerably and improved the ease of use. It seems prudent to me, however, just to use the safer drug.

HMOs mandate the use of Tagamet because of the price differential. For young people taking no other drugs, it is probably all right, but if other drugs or older age is a factor, HMO doctors should have the option of using Zantac or one of the others like it (Pepcid, Axid).

Tagamet, Zantac, and Pepcid were once available only by prescription, but they have followed another trend—the availability of more and more drugs over-the-counter without a prescription. Prescriptions provide safety for patients because they are regulated by doctors. Adverse medication interactions cause a huge number of negative effects and even deaths each year, and these interactions may become more common now that the drugs are available without a prescription.

While on the whole the benefits of most drugs outweigh the risks, the obvious principle is to use any drug only when clearly needed and worth more than the risk, and to do so very carefully with full knowledge and understanding of how to use it. For example, if a consumer buys Tagamet over the counter and takes it while on certain drugs for anticoagulation, heart disease, epilepsy, and psychiatric problems, significant adverse effects may occur, as noted in the PDR. Furthermore, taking any of the antacid drugs over-the-counter without consulting a physician may obscure but not cure a more serious disease such as cancer or complications of severe acid disorders.

Without training and education, how can consumers make properly informed decisions? Obviously, they cannot. When a doctor prescribes a drug properly, it is on the basis of a careful evaluation of the patient, many factors are taken into account, and the prescription is accompanied by careful explanation as to correct use, precautions, and what to watch out for. Good doctors learn about the many recent drugs by studying FDA information and leading medical journals.

If a doctor prescribes a drug, any adverse event is subject to scrutiny and censure if appropriate. If a consumer buys a drug and misuses it, there is no liability for the drug company or the legislators and regulators who permitted its nonprescription use. On the other hand, over-the-counter drugs are convenient for patients, increase patients' control of their own lives, and save the cost of seeing a doctor to get a prescription. It is a balance of pros and cons that deserves continual and careful reevaluation.

I believe there are serious issues to be resolved concerning drug prices, marketing, and research, but we must be very careful *how* we address these issues. Our pharmaceutical industry is both one of the jewels of our economy and an invaluable source of lifesaving treatments. We do *not* want to hinder its creativity and enterprise.

Staff and Research Cutbacks

In the past, "proprietary" hospitals had a terrible reputation. Proprietary hospitals were usually small, local hospitals operated for profit, whereas most hospitals were nonprofit, usually termed "voluntary." Proprietaries were usually not associated with medical schools, had few American-trained housestaff, if any, and often operated far out of touch with mainstream medicine. University hospitals were regularly called upon to salvage disasters.

A doctor named Thomas Frist Jr., along with a few others, transformed this situation as he and his associates formed companies that bought hospitals, both proprietary and voluntary, and converted them into units of a gigantic, for-profit, public company. The idea was, as with managed care, to bring modern business methods to the allegedly quaint, antiquated hospital business. It was thought that patients and businesspersons would both profit. In practice, however, only the owners benefited, at the expense of patients who had to spend much more time at home in pain and discomfort caring for themselves since patients were sent home sooner with less time to recuperate in the hospital where they would have support and care.

The hospital conversions did improve a few marginal hospitals, but, far more often, conversion degraded care while costing *more!* For-profit hospitals impose the stiff overhead of paying for the managed care company's profit and higher administrative cost. Medicare imposes limits similar to those of for-profit hospitals for the patients they cover and managed care restrictions tighten the noose even further. Voluntary hospitals are suffering from the competition but will find ways to remain profitable (just listen to your radio and TV for their commercials), but as in every case of cost-cutting, the patients and doctors will pay the price.

Hospitals are very large enterprises. Some are part of major medical centers with a medical school and many specialty hospitals on the same campus as the general hospital. A medical center is a magical place. It attracts the finest clinicians, researchers, and educators. It provides the highest quality care; carries out enormous volumes of research; and educates and trains doctors, nurses, and other health professionals. The center maintains contact with similar centers all over the world and there is an active interchange in this country and abroad.

Size is an advantage up to a point. Large centers with between 500 and 1,500 beds have the income to finance such an operation. They are able to support an extraordinary array of services and with few exceptions are the only places that can afford to pay attention to rare diseases and otherwise neglected problems.

Medical centers with medical schools develop traditions of very high standards. Though the medical center is huge, each service is still of a limited, manageable size so that personal, individualized care is not sacrificed. This is aided further by the large core of students and housestaff who bring the enthusiasm of youth and the dedication to learning their skills. These students and trainees add much greater value than they cost in inexperience, and they are closely supervised by senior doctors.

These hospitals made a lot of money even though they were non-profit and they didn't have to pay taxes. They charged excessive prices for insured patients because they needed excess funds to pay for the housestaff, the education of new doctors and paraprofessionals, and to pay for all the uninsured patients for whom they were the port of last resort. This was a poor, indirect, but necessary way to finance these important needs. If insurance companies now decline to contribute to these costs, will taxpayers be willing to pay higher taxes to do so? If insurers are held responsible, it will mean higher premiums, so one way or another, someone has to pay to staff hospitals with doctors, train new doctors, support research, and pay for the care of those who cannot pay their own bills.

All that changed with the growth of Medicare restrictions, managed care, and large hospital corporations, which gutted much of what makes these national treasures great.

First, Medicare put a maximum on what they would pay for a diagnosis requiring admission. A specified amount was allowed for a heart attack and a different amount for breast cancer surgery. Because people often have multiple diagnoses, DRGs (Diagnosis Related Groups) were developed. Utilization committees monitored admissions and discharges to ensure that DRGs stayed within the cost limit. A dance of strategy in coding had come to the hospitals, because the diagnosis and procedure codes determine DRG classification and thus reimbursement.

Then Medicare began to cut back on funding. Patients had to be discharged more quickly. This led to a glut of beds and more losses for the hospitals, since beds cost money even when they are empty, because they must be maintained to be available when needed. When managed care became powerful enough, it was able to forcefully extract punishing discounts from the hospitals that were not part of managed care companies already, while imposing ever greater administrative costs. Local hospitals that did not comply with managed care were often forced out of business as the managed care companies kept their patients away.

The hospital corporations, like the largest, Columbia/HCA, based on Dr. Frist's original company, began a massive acquisition of hospitals and the practices of the doctors associated with them. The remaining independent hospitals were forced to merge into huge alliances with far-flung affiliates. Strict cost controls were imposed leading to the reduction of nursing staffs by more than 25 percent.

Nurses are extraordinary people: their job is backbreaking, messy, highly demanding, and stressful. It pays little compared to its demands. Someone can only be a nurse out of absolute dedication and the joy of helping people in their time of greatest need.

It is disgraceful that the cost-cutters have reduced nursing staffs to levels that force the nurses to double their work and to suffer the agony of being forced to serve more people than they can properly handle. The nurses feel strongly that overwork directly increases errors (such as incorrect medication) and decreases quality of care. What is worse, hospitals are achieving these reductions by substituting minimally trained, lower-level workers who may have as little as a high school education and a few weeks' training.

If it were you in that hospital bed, who do you want to answer the call—a nurse with years of schooling, training, and experience or a high school graduate with a few weeks of instruction? Do you want a nurse who can spend time with you, hear your problems, and give you comfort, or a harried, overloaded, and exhausted aide who grouchily comes to your door?

Of equal import is the threat to education and research that the hospitals used to fund. The next generation of doctors will be shaped by today's education. How long can the great centers of learning and research maintain levels against the continuing cutbacks? Some alternative funding will be needed, as we discussed. Do you want your future doctors to be trained to work in a managed care world? They are right now. A whole generation of doctors will never have experienced the kind of medical care described in chapter 2.

Undermining the funding of research will deny ourselves all the remarkable advances that could be coming from university research centers. Private industry, as valuable as such companies are, just cannot substitute because university research can operate more freely than research geared toward the specific, narrower goals appropriate to a corporation. The federal government has increased funding to the National Institutes of Health, but how long will that continue? There will be a political limit of funding that may stop short of compensating for what has been lost.

Where will the uninsured go if the nonprofit hospitals disappear or lose the funds to pay for care of the uninsured? What will we say to the uninsured mother of a sick child who can no longer find a hospital that will help her?

MEDICARE AND MEDICAID

Some years ago, in New York State, someone in Albany decided to do something about the few doctors who were cheating Medicaid. These crooks were seeing one hundred patients per day and performing endless unnecessary tests to boost their income, to the tune of millions per year. In government-think, if a few citizens are doing something wrong, pass a law that punishes everybody to make sure you get every last one of the bad guys.

The politicians in Albany decided that they would make sure that their Medicaid clients did not visit private doctors, only clinics. They set the reimbursement rates in the range of $93 per visit to a clinic, $8 per visit to a doctor, and $4 for a doctor's hospital visit. (These amounts vary a little over time and by locality.) Few if any good doctors can afford to see Medicaid patients at these rates, which are far below what it costs to run an office. In New York it can cost as much as $100 to $200 per hour to run a medical office.

The poor and disabled need the protection and helping hand of the government wherever communities fail them. Major science projects and research are too large for local assistance. But government should not be managing our daily lives, invading our privacy, or deciding our health care for us. Obviously there are functions that only states and the federal government can do, but central planning of local care may hurt more than it helps. Thomas Jefferson was right: That government rules best which rules the least. When it comes to our private lives, the government should be almost imperceptibly involved.

Medicare and Medicaid cost a great deal of money, as do the veterans' health system and other government health facilities. We will discuss in the last chapter how that money might be better used.

When doctors have to answer to the government, the problem is different than the financial conflict of interest that occurs with managed care. The doctor still has divided loyalties, but in this case, the pressure to limit your care is from the punitively heavy hand of Uncle Sam and the state governments. As I mentioned earlier, Medicare should at least be only for the needy. Now it is a welfare program for the rich as well. If those who could afford their own insurance were taken off the government dole, which is what the Medicare subsidy really is, there would be more money to more adequately fund the care of those who truly need financial support.

ALTERNATIVE CARE

"Alternative care" is a euphemism for unproven remedies that are outside of the medical mainstream. These treatments are sometimes called "natural," which then allows them to slip through legal loopholes and escape the jurisdiction of the Food and Drug Administration. If a drug is labeled "natural," it escapes FDA jurisdiction. All food extracts, vitamins, and the like, when given with promise of a beneficial effect are, by definition, drugs, but unfortunately, not according to Congress's definition. Thus, they can be sold to you with *no* proof that they work or that they are safe. Serious injuries have sometimes resulted. Natural remedies can also raise false hopes, a cruel thing to do to people in need. They may deter people from treatments that are more likely to help. They may put people through unnecessary discomfort and even cause death.

People who just wanted a good night's sleep bought L-tryptophan, a synthetic version of an amino acid in the body, touted as a good sleep aide. At least thirty died from a rare disorder called eosinophilia-myalgia syndrome. Thousands more were badly injured but survived.[5] Sleep experts I asked felt L-tryptophan was ineffective as a sleep aid, so people took a significant risk for little if any value. The numbers were so great that the drug was removed from the market.

A recent review in the *American Journal of Medicine* details an alarming list of hazards from herbal remedies, medicines made from naturally occurring plant products or other substances, as opposed to drugs synthesized to be used as treatments.

- Young people died trying ephedrine-containing compounds purchased in health food stores. The compounds sold as mood enhancers were used by youths to get high.
- Ginseng has caused brain inflammation and severe mood disturbances. There are many claims for ginseng which I cannot easily cite as they vary from author to author, something which is true of all these remedies.
- Many "natural remedies" have caused severe rashes or allergic reactions as well as serious drug interactions.
- Many of the remedies, including chaparral, germander, comfrey, and pennyroyal, for all of which there are many shifting, unproven claims of benefit, cause severe liver damage.
- Guar gum has caused severe intestinal obstruction.

- Many remedies are contaminated with lead, mercury, arsenic, steroids, and a host of other toxic substances.[6]

The list goes on and on.

If I walked into my backyard and scooped up some dirt, put it in a fancy bottle, and said it was a natural substance that would impart the spirit of Gaia to give you well-being, there is nothing any authority could do to stop me from selling it.

Alternative care proponents claim that more Americans now visit homeopaths and other such practitioners than visit primary care doctors, but such self-serving statistics are very suspect. The newest approach is to mix real medicine concepts with unproven alternative medicine ideas to give the alternatives legitimacy. It is called "complementary" or "integrative" medicine, but I believe that the problems of unproven treatments are not remedied by mixing them with mainstream medicine concepts.

The rising economic and political power of alternative medicine has propelled legal and academic recognition of these newly named variants. If this brings regulation and legitimate testing of claims and products, that may at least reduce the risks and verify any effectiveness they may have.

I would urge that we invest heavily in investigating folk remedies that have been used for generations. Many worthwhile treatments have been discovered that way, such as digitalis, used for heart disease, and curare, which was a valuable drug in surgery in earlier days. Claims made for herbs and plants should be studied if they have any legitimate history. If St. John's wort, claimed to be an effective treatment for anxiety and depression, has something good, let's find it.

What we should not do is experiment on people without their knowing it, taking advantage of the vulnerability we all have when it comes to our health and well being. When you give or sell someone something that has never been adequately tested with a promise of some result, you are experimenting. It is as if you went out into the woods with no knowledge of mushrooms and picked some, hoping they were not a poisonous variety.

We should not make promises and expose people to something that has not been proven safe and effective.

Mainstream treatments cause many adverse effects. This is a major problem, but, as we have discussed, there is always risk in trying to help. The difference is that in mainstream medicine, billions of dollars and thousands of hours of research are expended to be as sure as possible that treatments are reasonably effective and safe. When they have been cleared to be used, they are employed by highly skilled professionals for specific indications and then monitored closely and carefully. None of this is done for alternative treatments.

When you go to a health food store or order by mail or take something from a well-intentioned friend, you are acting on belief, not science or fact. Although belief is great for religion and politics, it has no place in finding ways to safely make you healthier.

Managed care has encouraged use of alternative medicine in two ways. First, by destroying the doctor-patient relationship and stealing the time doctors should have with patients, it has pushed people into the arms of those who spend time and listen and make promises. Second, some managed care companies, such as Oxford Health Plans, have added alternative medicine providers to their networks and reimburse for their services and products. This may be an effort to meet subscribers' desire for these services, but I believe it may also be a way of saving money by steering customers to less expensive alternative providers, thus saving the companies the expense of seeing physicians.

If alternative remedies are as worthless as so many of them seem, then consider how much of our precious resources we are diverting from legitimate care.

NOTES

1. Michael L. Millenson, *Demanding Medical Excellence* (Chicago: University of Chicago Press, 1997).

2. A. Z. Carr, "Can an Executive Afford a Conscience?" in *Ethics in Practice,* ed. K. R. Andrew (Boston: Harvard Business School Press, 1989), pp. 26–34.

3. Stephanie Stapleton, "Drug Recalls Raise Questions about FDA Drug Approvals," *American Medical News* 41 (August 17, 1998): 57–59.

4. George Anders, *Health against Wealth, HMOs and the Breakdown of Medical Trust* (New York: Houghton Mifflin, 1996): 50–53.

5. National Eosinophilia-myalgia Syndrome Network, http://www.nemsn.org/ems/html.

6. Edzard Ernst, "Harmless Herbs? A Review of the Recent Literature," *American Journal of Medicine* 104 (February 1998): 170–78.

12

Issues

That which enters the mind through reason can be corrected. That which is admitted through faith, hardly ever.

—Santiago Ramón y Cajal

Each of us must make informed decisions, not just about our own health care, but equally importantly, how we as citizens will design the systems under which we all must live. It is time for all of us to participate in the debate. You are currently living under a health care system created by business and government. Business profit and government cost containment motivate them, perhaps more than your welfare. How can we decide our own fate if we do not understand the forces at work and the issues we must decide?

From the rugged individualists who created a unique society and conquered a wild continent we have become a nation of sheep so preoccupied with daily minutiae that we have abdicated our personal responsibility. We are paying a high price as a small segment of society is gaining enormous power and wealth at the expense of the many.

We have been discussing how this is occurring in health care. The health you lose may be your own. We should all wake up, pay attention, and take back what is rightfully ours. It is not too late.

What follows are some of the issues all of us should understand and of which you should form your own opinions. The discussions are brief to keep them accessible, but I hope they stimulate heated debates that will illuminate and create.

Most of these issues are not peculiar to managed care. They are issues society has always faced and will continue to struggle with. The difference with managed care is that profit motives of those far removed from direct patient care change the equations of decision.

IS MANAGED CARE ETHICALLY AND MORALLY UNACCEPTABLE? I BELIEVE IT IS.

- It forces the doctor to serve two masters.
- It is fee splitting.
- It cuts so close to the bare minimum or below that it puts patients at risk.
- It invades patients' privacy.
- It steals the time essential to good care.
- It forces a particular form of treatment instead of what may be right for the individual.
- It imposes cookbook care instead of allowing care tailored to the individual needs of each patient.
- It subverts informed consent.
- It purports to cover you for the care your doctor feels you need, but denies that care using non-doctors or doctors with conflicts of interest who do not even see you. In other words, it promises comprehensive care but denies it arbitrarily.
- It promises quality, but, by its very nature, it degrades quality care.
- It substitutes lesser-trained practitioners for fully qualified doctors.
- It destroys the doctor-patient relationship.

These problems cannot be fixed—I believe they are inherent to the very nature of managed care. We can have ethical care or we can have managed care, but we cannot have both.

SHOULD WE PROVIDE HEALTH CARE INSURANCE FOR EVERYONE?

Uwe Reinhardt, James Madison Professor of Political Economy at Princeton University, is a leading philosopher on health care economics. He has posed this question:

> As a matter of national policy, and to the extent that a nation's health system can make it possible, should the child of a poor American family have the same chance of avoiding preventable illness or of being cured from a given illness as does the child of a rich family?[1]

One would think that in America on the brink of a new millennium, this question would have been answered long ago. As he notes, there are more than ten million children not covered by health insurance and millions more whose coverage is inadequate. Many of these children suffer real injury because of their lack of access to decent care. Over 30 million adults are also uncovered, often at a considerable health cost as well.

Not only do children of lower economic levels not have equal access to basic, decent care, nothing is being done about it because many in positions of power do not feel any obligation for government to expend funds on those who cannot purchase their own insurance.

Reinhardt, in his essay "Wanted—A Clearly Articulated Social Ethic for American Health Care" and in subsequent letters that appeared in the *Journal of the American Medical Association,* in effect, debates an author named Richard Epstein and also refers to work by Milton Friedman of the very conservative Chicago School of Economics.[2] An esoteric debate between ivory tower economists may seem of little interest to our everyday lives, but, unfortunately, these opinions directly affect the care that you receive in your doctor's office, so we must pay close attention. I will use this debate as a way of discussing some critical issues we must confront.

Conservative economists like Epstein and Friedman express the views of like-minded members of Congress. They believe in the trickle-down theory, the general idea of which is that to the extent that capitalism is allowed unfettered growth, the most successful members of society will profit, using their energy and resources to invest in new business and in other segments of the economy. That should redound to the benefit of the less entrepreneurial by the creation of jobs and the general elevation of wealth. Epstein, in a letter commentary on Rheinhardt's article, argues that the same will hold true for health care.

There is certainly validity to the ability of capitalism to create a healthy economy that benefits all, but whether enough crumbs trickle down is another matter. Few of us "average Joes" benefit from the many government subsidies available to the rich, for example. Epstein also correctly notes that government programs are often inefficient and ineffective. He is way off base, however, when he offers the popular conservative elitist line that government beneficence discourages initiative by coddling the poor and being overprotective. He and others who believe this are confusing the adverse effects of *some* welfare programs with the provision of essential health needs.

Perhaps those who believe this should have the opportunity to experience life as an unemployed inner city mother with little hope of a job, or as a homeless Vietnam veteran unable to escape the ravaging aftereffects of that awful war, or as a laid-off, downsized, blue-collar family man who sees his family thrown out into the street because his services are no longer needed by a large corporation whose executives receive multimillion dollar salaries.

Some people are uninsured by choice, but far more are in that position unwillingly—they simply cannot afford the cost of health insurance. The conservatives counter that uninsured does not necessarily mean untreated, since health care is still available—at the person's own expense.

The few choices for uninsured people who are not rich include the charity of doctors and the hospital emergency room. I have always treated people according to their means and I have given my share of free care as well—most doctors I know do the same. But it is absurd to think that the needs of the uninsured can or should be met in this way. The second recourse, the emergency room, is fine if you are suffering a grievous *emergency*, but is an absurd way to deliver routine care. Patients who have nowhere to go for care except the emergency room delay treatment until it becomes far more expensive and difficult, and in an emergency room, it is handled superficially. Emergency rooms are designed, naturally enough, for *emergencies*. ERs should not turn away any patient they have not ensured is safe to do so, so by default they become the primary caretaker for many people who do not have emergencies, but they are not equipped to handle that role satisfactorily. They could not remain emergency rooms if they turn themselves into properly equipped primary care clinics.

It is not the fault of the doctors or the hospital—emergency rooms were never intended for that purpose. Our emergency rooms are now so overloaded that they are severely impaired in their ability to handle true emergencies and the whole process adds an enormous excess cost to health care.

The third resource for the uninsured is discounted clinic care in municipal hospitals, which are already so overcrowded that it is nearly impossible for them to deliver good care.

Moreover, under managed care and for-profit hospital takeovers, the number of hospitals that will even be able to treat uninsured patients is shrinking fast. The profits from full-pay patients that they formerly used for the poor have dried up to nothing by the cost-cutting effects of managed care and profit-driven hospital corporations.

For-profit care is only for healthy people with enough money. The government chooses to favor only the poorest of the poor. The large group that falls between Medicaid poverty and middle class is left out in the cold, literally. Congress is torn between the liberal desire to help the less well off and its reluctance to increase taxes on the majority to pay for it.

The conservative economists can pontificate all they want, but our country needs a soul as much as it needs wealth, it needs decency as much as it needs democracy, it needs fairness as much as it needs capitalism's free enterprise. We do not want to go the way of ancient Rome, wealthy in material goods, impoverished in soul, weakened until finally destroyed by our own excesses.

I believe that we can craft a free-enterprise, capitalistic, entrepreneurial, successful society in which some mechanisms exist to ensure that all of us have an equal chance and a decent basic standard of living. Within such a society, we must decide if all of us will have *reasonable* opportunity for a decent standard of living, and, particularly, access to decent health care. I do not see how we can permit our fellow citizens to suffer unnecessary damage to their health. These are our neighbors and they include children, families, elderly people, and the most vulnerable among us.

EQUAL CARE OR EQUAL ACCESS?

The measure of our society is not what wealth we accumulate but how well we provide for the least fortunate among us. Doctors see the misery of deprivation in all its intensity. What should compel us to be doctors should equally drive us to do what we can to ensure that no one suffers needlessly. That does *not* mean that every member of society must be equal. Even if such a goal were possible, what a dull life it would be, devoid of variety, ambitions, goals, dreams, and passions curtailed by the imposition of conformity. The Russian experiment with communism proved conclusively that human nature is contrary to enforced egalitarianism. Communism failed miserably in almost every country that tried it and the few remaining are likely destined for the same fate.

This raises a crucial question. If we should enforce equal health care, why stop at that, why not make everyone equal in everything? Where *do* we draw the line of creating equality by government decree?

Society *cannot* successfully enforce equality, even if it were the right thing to do. Trying to create a false equality only distorts society and creates more problems than it helps. We should by all means make a college education equally available to every child, but to attempt to use government power to make every college experience equal would not only be futile, it would destroy great institutions like Princeton University at little benefit to the lesser colleges or to society. The same is true for medicine, as we shall discuss below.

I believe unequivocally that every American should have the right to basic, decent medical care. I do *not* believe that we must all have the same level of health care, no more than I believe that we should all have the same income, the same size house, or the same education.

We all have the right to life, liberty, and the *pursuit* of happiness. Nowhere is it mandated that the government should guarantee that we all have the same amount of quality of everything.

Health care *is* different. Without health, nothing else matters. What good are wealth and power for a man whose memory has been destroyed though Alzheimer's? What good does achieving the height of business success do when cancer strikes at a young age? What good does it do a great athlete to reach the pinnacle of human physical ability only to have his heart physically betray him?

The famous make headlines, but illness and disability can rob any one of us of our lives, our families, our dreams. When you hear the doctor tell you the lump is cancer, or you feel that terrible pressure in your chest, or suddenly you cannot speak or use half of your body, all of your daily life becomes insignificant as you face the threat to your very existence. It would be wonderful *if* we could achieve perfect health care for all, but such a thing is impossible.

The cry of the 1990s is that we have limited resources and that we must determine how best to allocate them. We will discuss later just how much of our resources we should devote to health care, but first we must discuss the "distribution" issue, as economists might phrase it. In other words, *who gets what?*

If we agree that we have limited resources, then there are several ways we could allocate them. One way is what we do now: Today, the rich have all the health care possible at insignificant cost for them, but nevertheless made even more affordable by the tax deductibility of health insurance and medical costs, a significant benefit at higher tax brackets. The middle class *had* good health care at somewhat high cost before managed care. Since managed care, they now have mediocre to barely adequate care at too high a cost. The lowest income groups have Medicaid and Medicare, which provide poor to barely adequate care. The uninsured are the worst off. They have only emergency room or clinic care, which is woefully inadequate.

Another way is to ensure that every person is financially equal. At present, some have more and some have less. To achieve equality would mean that we either add more money to bring the "have-lesses" up to the level of the "have-mores," or, we take away from the have-mores to give to the have-lesses. If we say we cannot spend any more, the only choice would be to take from the haves to give to the have-nots.

Suppose that we do the latter, taking from those who have more to finance the care of those who have less. We could do this by creating a price-controlled system, like Medicare, that would apply to every citizen and which would be financed by a progressive tax, unlike Medicare, which is a regressive tax.* This would give everyone equal care and its cost would be proportionally higher for the wealthy.

This is a so-called single-payer plan and it has many supporters. They point to other countries as examples, since essentially every other country in the world uses some variant of a single-payer plan. According to proponents, the rest of the world not only has a fairer system, but one that delivers better health care at a fraction of the cost that we expend.

Now this sounds great: inexpensive, high-quality health care delivered equally to all, funded by those who can well afford it. If you believe that this utopia is possible in our country, think again. Many of those who are opposed to managed care are in favor of the single-payer plan. However, the majority of Americans are "have-mores," though not many are "have-enoughs." They are not-enoughs, which means that they have basic care, but are at significant risk if they need care beyond the minimum because managed care is so restrictive. If we have to take from them to finance the have-lesses, most of the money will come from these at-risk middle-class Americans. There are many more of them than there are rich people. *Therefore, in effect, we would be lowering the level of care of the many, who are already marginal, to benefit the few.* That makes no sense to me.

How else could we do it? Well, there are always those overpaid doctors. They have made too much for too long, so let us just issue a gov-

---

*A progressive tax takes an increasingly higher percentage of income as income goes up. A regressive tax takes the same percentage of tax from all income levels. Regressive taxes are much harder on the lower end, because even though the percentage paid is the same, the proportion of the person's total income used is much higher for the low end than for the high end. In other words, if a poor man pays $100 in tax, that is a major expense; if a wealthy person pays $1,000, it is easily affordable.

ernment decree that anyone who wants to practice medicine in America must become a government employee and earn what the government thinks is enough for them.

Let us say that we succeed and everyone has single-payer health coverage. So now we have, all of a sudden, more than 40 million more Americans who are free to go see doctors just like everyone else. They will have to compete with all the people who have had access all along. *All* Americans would then have to seek care from a conscripted army of former professionals who have been forced into government service at low pay. At least no one will get any care better than that given to someone else. We will all get equally bad care but we will all be equal.

And we will still be spending too much money. There is just not enough money to save by reducing doctors' incomes to pay for the care of 40 million more people. And if you did this would medical schools be overflowing with applicants? Furthermore, none of this solves the problems that plague the rest of the system.

Medicaid and Medicare, which right now are single-payer plans for specific groups, have given us hints of the perils of such a system. Imagine if one becomes universal.

Let us just review where we stand. Let us assume that most Americans would favor helping those who are uninsured, so that their fellow citizens and those 10 million children would not continue to suffer unnecessary poor health. Whether our generous citizens would be willing to pay the cost in the form of substantially higher taxes is another story, but for now let us make the very risky assumption that they would. A single-payer system would accomplish the goal of health care for all by (1) lowering the quality of care for the population as a whole; (2) conscripting and forcing into lower income the very people needed to enthusiastically provide the care that is required; (3) require substantially higher cost in taxes; and (4) place the health and most private information of the American people squarely into the hands of government bureaucrats.

Knowing how well the government handles important matters, would you want such a system? Perhaps it is not surprising that Americans rejected the Clinton health care initiative and remain skeptical of huge, expensive government programs involving their health and privacy.

Each of us must begin to consider that if we believe in providing decent basic care for the least able of us, are we willing to pay for it? We must decide if we are going to lower the quality of care for the many in order to provide for those less able to provide for themselves or if we are willing to spend more to help them.

RATIONING—WHO DECIDES HOW MUCH HEALTH CARE YOU GET

"We cannot ration health," many might say. Not only can we, we do it all the time. When I see a patient for a comprehensive check-up, there are certain tests that are indicated by the exam or history to rule out a disease. There are other tests that can be done that will look for problems so early that there is not yet any outward sign to suggest the need. For example, pernicious anemia, a type of Vitamin B_{12} deficiency, was once a common condition in elderly people that presented symptoms of anemia, mental changes, beefy red tongue, burning nerve pains, odd sensations in the arms and legs called paresthesias, and eventually paralysis and dementia. Partly due to better care and partly for reasons unknown, severe cases became uncommon and B_{12} testing was often forgotten. Then research showed that B_{12} deficiency is still occurring in people as young as forty, particularly women, though it is showing itself in less obvious ways. Sometimes the only symptoms are paresthesias or subtle memory loss. It also is still common among older people and is one of the reversible causes of memory loss and thus vital to rule out before diagnosing an irreversible disease like Alzheimer's. Since permanent nerve and memory damage can result before the disease is recognized, and since it is easily treatable, I think screening people over forty for B_{12} makes sense, but it is seldom recognized by managed care insurance companies as a reimbursable screening test.

Thus, I ask my patients if they would want to have the test done by the outside lab at their own expense (if they do not have a diagnosis that the insurance company would accept). Some decide to get the test, others do not. Those who do not are rationing their own funds, deciding where to save money to apply to other expenses.

Medicare will probably not pay for the test as a screening test because they are rationing their limited funds and have decided that screening tests like this take a lower priority than other needs. They would likely argue that it costs too much to test everyone to find too few people who would benefit. Managed care companies will find even more reasons to decline to pay for the test.

Managed care is supposed to ration to enhance quality by shifting funds from wasteful or less important uses to higher-quality interventions. In practice, it rations almost entirely to enhance profit. Shifting money into your own pockets is not rationing.

Even Paul Ellwood, the father of managed care, admits that, so far, managed care decisions are based only on cost and profit, though he remains ever optimistic that companies will begin to compete over quality.[3] I won't hold my breath waiting.

Rationing is a tough subject. None of us wants to think that we are rationing, but that is the reality. If needs exceed resources, we must choose which needs to meet. If a group of survivors of a shipwreck are in a lifeboat, starving after days at sea, food and water almost gone, how do they decide who shall live and who shall die? Do they simply feed the sickest or do they decide whether to save the six-year-old versus the sixty-year-old? What if two six-year-olds are dying? Or do the strongest simply take from the weakest? Such horrible choices are almost unbearable examples of rationing. In such cases, there is no way to evade the reality of what you are doing and the issue is concrete.

Governments must also ration. The United States owes trillions of dollars, and projections suggest that Social Security and Medicare will run out of money at some point in the future. The Medicare and Social Security trust funds contain only IOUs from the government to itself. The actual money has been lent out in the form of bonds. The funds collect interest, but it's just more money that the government owes itself. Projections are risky, as we noted earlier, but there are many debates now as to how to forestall that future risk.

Payroll taxes, interest, and premiums pay Medicare benefits. As the baby boomers age and enter eligibility for Medicare, their needs will exceed what the remaining workforce can pay under current levels. That means either increased taxes or decreased benefits or both. If we do neither, then we will have to borrow more, thus further increasing the national debt. If the economy falters, that reduces income to Medicare, creating a vicious cycle.

To counter this, Medicare is attempting to bring patients under managed care and is trying other variations as well. It is also cutting back on benefits indirectly by creating ever-greater bureaucratic hurdles for doctors. The ugly "R" word (rationing) is being whispered around the halls of government, but very quietly, lest the AARP hear it.

Physicians are in the unenviable position of being right on the firing line of rationing decisions imposed by managed care, the government, and patients. Patients all want the best medical care at minimal cost. Managed care wants less spent so it can maximize its profits and please investors. The government does not want to run out of money. And politicians know that whatever they do, they do not want to raise taxes and reduce their chances for reelection.

A doctor's primary responsibility is to the patient sitting in his office at that moment. His duty to that patient is to mobilize all that modern medicine can offer to solve that patient's problem, within the patient's means and according to the patient's wishes. If every doctor does this for every patient, then society must decide how to provide the money needed to care for 265 million Americans without taking too much from other needs.

The decisions physicians face can be very direct. Consider heart transplants. There are never enough hearts to treat all who need them. Each heart allocated to one patient is a death sentence to another patient who remains on the waiting list.

In England, similar choices must be made on a larger scale. The government has imposed an absolute cap on total health spending and set specific limits in some areas, such as transplants. English doctors face choices every day: Does this patient need this procedure or should it be preserved for someone else? If I spend too much on this patient, who will go without something else? In the English system, such decisions have no direct bearing on the doctor's income, so the doctor is really acting as a disinterested mediator between individual patient needs and society's limits.[4] The absence of personal financial motive makes the process fairer, but it deprives the patient of the doctor's full devotion to the patient's own care since the doctor is serving two masters.

Capitated managed care contracts force doctors to make continual rationing decisions, but here the doctor faces a powerful conflict between decisions that benefit the doctor financially versus those for the patient's benefit.

One way to ration is for society to impose external limits on specific items. This has been done in Oregon where the state's Medicaid program has instituted a unique approach never tried elsewhere. Called the Oregon Basic Health Services Program, it openly and proudly rations health care for Medicaid patients, using the word "rationing" forthrightly.[5] The plan, after long deliberation, established a list of 709 paired medical conditions and treatments ranked according to clinical effectiveness, cost, and social importance. Plan organizers decided to pay for the top 587 items on the list. Any item below that would not be available to poor patients except at their own expense.*

The initial ranking was seriously flawed, putting the capping of teeth above an appendectomy or ranking a vasectomy higher than

---

*The plan involved mandates for insurance for other groups and other aspects beyond our scope here.

treating infertility. These were revised and made somewhat more reasonable, but true prioritizing is virtually impossible.

Compressing 10,000 diagnoses into 709 procedures is an absurd enterprise. Attempting to assign numeric values for ranking purposes to concepts as unmeasurable as fairness, justice, and need is the height of arrogance. Most of all, it precludes the very nature of medical care, the tailoring of care to the specific needs of each patient.

The plan is a committee product (recall in chapter 7 our previous discussion of the dangers of committee-itis) that imposes other people's moral judgments on an entire segment of the population. It also singles out the most vulnerable population, the poor, and exempts the rest of society from sacrificing anything. Oregon deserves an E for effort, an F for execution, and an A for dealing with rationing directly and honestly instead of secretly and hypocritically as most of America does.

External rationing by society tells doctors what to ration, how to do so, and who gets what. This would appear to take the physician off the hook, but it does not. Such plans violate the basic requirement that doctors tailor their care to the specific needs of the patients who are their responsibility. Doctors would be forced either to try to bend the external limitations to their patients' needs or to violate their own obligation to do the best for their patients in order to adhere to the higher power of the system.

Such external rationing is the "it's not my job" or the "I am just obeying orders" excuse. It *is* the doctor's job and no outside agency can relieve the doctor of the moral and professional obligation to do what is right for the patient. What is right for the patient does not mean pushing for every possible benefit regardless of reason or need. It means exercising good judgment to give good care for that patient's unique needs.

Another way to ration would be the physician carrying out what is known as bedside rationing. In this case, the doctor decides when and what care to limit for the greater societal good. Should the doctor refer this patient for a liver transplant or reserve that scarce, precious organ for someone who is a better candidate? Should he screen this patient for B_{12} deficiency, or save those dollars so that the general funds are not depleted? Again, our long-suffering physician is put in a difficult bind between his obligation as physician and his position of power in handling society's resources. Every physician should do this routinely with every decision up to a point. We all have an obligation to society to use shared resources wisely.

What should be beyond the purview of the physician is to attempt to solve the economic problems of the whole by sacrificing important care for the individual to whom the physician is primarily responsible. In other words, both doctor and patient should be sensible, but neither should be responsible for solving society's larger funding problems.

Some authors have discussed a variant on this, what could be termed surrogate rationing—the doctor acts as surrogate for what he *presumes* the patient would decide.[6] The idea is that the physician should know what the patient would want and act accordingly. For example, if the doctor thinks that a patient who pays a portion of the cost of medicines would choose a cheaper, less effective drug if it meant lower cost to the patients, the doctor would prescribe the cheaper drug as long as it was reasonably acceptable. In another case, the doctor may surmise that a patient would choose to avoid an expensive and unpleasant procedure and accept an inferior result without it and thus not recommend the procedure. This concept is now being used to resolve ethical conflicts under managed care.

David Asch and Peter Ubel, in an article titled "Rationing by Any Other Name," take surrogate rationing a step further and describe various scenarios wherein the physician finds ways to justify choosing a cheaper test or treatment.[7] The physician has to find ways to rationalize that the chosen care, even if not the best care, is all right because it is in the patient's interest that costs be kept under control and thus premiums kept lower. This should not be the physician's role, nor should doctors surmise or assume what a patient would prefer.

The doctor should advise the patient about *all* of the available choices, and discuss the pros and cons, including managed care restraints if applicable, so that both can arrive at a mutually acceptable decision. As physicians, we are expert advisors to our patients, not their parents making choices for them.

A third way of rationing is to prearrange with the patient how much care will be given. Paying for liver transplants makes insurance policies much more expensive. Suppose each person is given a choice of signing a cheaper policy without transplant coverage or a more expensive one that includes it. Each patient would have to calculate for him- or herself or for their families the chance of needing a transplant versus the cost of having the right to one if needed.

Most people in good health who are not alcoholic would choose to forego the expensive coverage. Sounds perfect. The doctor has given the patient the choice, society is served, and care is tailored individually. Now suppose one of the nontransplant coverage patients, let's choose a thirty-year-old mother of three, contracts an aggressively virulent viral hepatitis A, goes rapidly downhill, and is near death. I saw such a case when I was a resident. The patient was a seventeen-year-old girl. The world's leading expert on the disease was an attending at the hospital and yet he could do nothing but stand by helplessly and watch her die in less than three weeks despite what little there was to do in 1969. Liver transplants were not available then.

So now what do you do about your young mother of three? "You did not buy insurance, so you pay with your life." Tell that to her three children. Can the community raise the money? Can the hospital afford to operate free? Some times the answer is no. Is the doctor off the hook just because the patient agreed ahead of time? No, the doctor must keep fighting to get the transplant up to the time of death.

Doctors should not ration, other than the obvious obligation not to employ unnecessary, wasteful, or counterproductive procedures, which is inherent in good care anyway. How, then, do we sensibly allocate limited resources? First, we ensure that the limits on resources for health care are not set too low. Second, we must recognize that whatever we do must be flexible and local. There are no clear answers, there are many sensible demands on the resources, and there is no way to lock in rules that would cover all of the nearly infinite permutations of interacting needs. Distant central authorities should not apply rigid rules to individual problems.

Flexibility is a double-edged sword. The hospital might opt to bend the rules for the young mother above, but that same hospital might feel no sympathy for a minority mother otherwise identical. Even without the prejudices that remain toxic within our society, our hearts may go out to a young mother, but not to a cranky fifty-year-old minimum wage earner. If there was only one liver, should it be given to the young mother, who neither smokes or drinks and has a whole family dependent on her survival, or to an alcoholic loner who will likely drink the new liver into failure as well? That is an easier decision. But if it is a nonprofit hospital forced nearly to bankruptcy by the predatory and monopolistic practices of a competing for-profit hospital, will giving the young mother the transplant free become the last straw leading to the closure of the only remaining nonprofit hospital?

None of these choices can be made in Washington or in the distant boardroom of a large corporation. Local elders should make these decisions locally, with flexibility and consultation with the local community. When free to do so, hospitals try to do just that, but their authority to do so may become increasingly limited by managed care and government policies.

Third, policies should be reviewed and revised continuously. There must be several levels of independent appeal, available promptly and with decisions made expeditiously. Delay in health care is a decision in itself.

Fourth, we should look for wisdom. Wisdom is fact and logic combined with experience and an active intelligence. Since medicine and environmental controls are lengthening lifespan, our society is aging. Yet, we are becoming an oligarchy of the young. Because our world is changing so fast technologically, financially, and globally, the general assumption is that only the young can understand the brave new world. So-called primitive societies, which were more "civilized" than we in some ways, endured and prospered for centuries because they valued the wisdom of their elders passed from generation to generation.

Rationing needs wisdom and experience. Society must set general limits and they must be applied locally with reason and compassion. The fewer committees and the fewer rules, the better.

FUTILE CARE

There comes a point where all treatment fails and there is nothing left to do. Modern medicine cannot cure everything. The dream is that someday we can, but then we will have another problem—where to put everyone.

In the past, when someone's time had come, the person stopped breathing and the heart stopped beating. Today, we can keep lungs pumping and hearts beating almost indefinitely, so a new definition of death has become necessary. Now, at least legally, death does not occur until a person is competently found to be "brain dead," for which certain specific neurological criteria must be met. A patient may not meet the criteria for brain death, yet never regain consciousness. If the person is completely unresponsive, the term "vegetative state" is used. Some patients may be at a slightly higher level, which is a coma. They may remain in that condition indefinitely. Patients in comas and even deeper levels of loss can be kept alive for what may be unlimited periods of time, but maintaining them is extremely expensive. The deeper the level of unconsciousness, the more bodily functions must be maintained artificially, and the more it costs.

The case of Karen Ann Quinlan brought these issues into public awareness and began to establish law.[8] Karen was a young woman who had lapsed into a coma, apparently from a combination of alcohol and tranquilizers, and was kept alive by an artificial respirator. Doctors reached the conclusion that she would never regain consciousness. Her family felt that it was immoral to maintain her in this hopeless state and that it was emotionally and financially impossible for them to go on. They requested that the hospital withdraw artificial life support and allow nature to take its course, whatever that might be. The doctors and the hospital refused on the grounds that it was against medical ethics. They felt that the obligation to preserve life outweighed the obligation to honor the patient's autonomy over his or her own life.

Karen's parents took their cause to court—eventually as high as the New Jersey Supreme Court. Prior to this landmark case, which remained prominently in the news throughout its long course, such requests were routinely refused—officially—by hospitals, doctors, and nursing homes, for several reasons. Religious objections by the doctor or hospital play a role, but the most prominent reason is that ending life, or even not prolonging it when such is still possible, is so contrary to the very being and soul of medicine that no doctor readily does so. Throughout the history of medicine doctors have been called upon by patients to relieve hopeless suffering by active means. Some doctors have done so quietly and others have never done so. When it was done, it was a quiet decision made by the doctor, the patient if possible, and the family, in privacy.

Another reason doctors are reluctant to act publicly is that, regardless of the request by the patient or those who have legal guardianship in the case of comatose patients, terminating life actively or discontinuing life-prolonging efforts raises the specter of malpractice or criminal prosecution for battery, murder, or assisted suicide. Few doctors felt they could take the chance that such a charge would be brought because there were no prior rulings that would adequately clarify their position.

The New Jersey Supreme Court in 1976 changed all that by ruling that the request to remove life support was valid for Karen Ann Quinlan; it did not violate medical ethics since there was no hope of recovery to a conscious state; to maintain her life was an imposition of a hopeless invasive treatment; and patients have the right to refuse treatment. The court specified that the doctors, the hospital, and the parents would be immune from legal action. If the hospital ethics committee agreed that her recovery was hopeless, Karen could be removed from the respirator. The respirator was removed and she lived for another ten years in a coma from which she never recovered.

Since that time, the issue has expanded to raise much broader questions: Can even food and water be withheld? Can a patient request a doctor end life by injection of an excessive dose of the morphine being administered for pain relief? Can a doctor assist a patient to commit suicide to end a life of medically hopeless pain and suffering? Dr. Jack Kevorkian has brought this issue into sharp focus for the public. The Netherlands allows such practice, and, in our country, Oregon has instituted just such a law.

The sovereignty of each person over his or her own life has come far from the days when suicide was illegal in most jurisdictions. I do not know how many such laws persist, but the courts and the field of ethics is coming to honor our right to ourselves as absolute and paramount. While common sense and any sensible understanding of the American ideal of individual freedom should make the right of personal sovereignty self-evident and incontrovertible, it raises as many painful moral issues as it solves.

The easiest to see are the religious objections of millions of Americans to whom suicide, assisted death, and such are anathema and totally contrary to their beliefs. We do not want to create unnecessary political divisions, nor to offend our fellow citizens thoughtlessly, but too many Americans died to preserve the rights guaranteed in the Constitution and the Bill of Rights, among which are the right to freedom of religion and for state and religion to be kept absolutely separate. While all Americans are free to exercise their religious beliefs in their own personal actions, should they decide for others?

This may seem far removed from medical economics, but in fact, it is a critical issue. Among the highest medical expense is the care in the last six months of life for patients with prolonged terminal illness. As I discussed in an earlier chapter, I suspect that the magnitude of this expense has been exaggerated for political purposes, but even so, it is still a major drain on resources.

The issue is, how long should support be given to someone whose case is hopeless and very expensive? Consider these cases:

A. A patient who may require prolonged and very expensive intensive care but who has a significant chance of recovery to a useful life. (We will discuss the definition of "useful" shortly.)
B. A patient with a serious illness who needs intensive, expensive care for a prolonged period but who will recover to have long periods of useful life of undeterminable duration.
C. A patient who has terminal cancer, was in intensive care for two weeks, seemingly comatose, known to have only a short time left, only to recover to have another six months of time very meaningful to him and his family.

D. A patient who is aware, able to talk briefly with family and friends, but unable to survive outside of intensive care.
E. A patient who is unconscious or mostly so, hopeless, requiring intensive care to survive.
F. A comatose or vegetative patient requiring intensive care, with no hope of recovery.
G. A patient like Karen Ann Quinlan, who survives without life support but requires maintenance care, which becomes very costly over time.

Consider, now, that you are sitting in your office in an imaginary country called Socialdom. You are the chairman of the rationing committee for the national health service, which is a nonprofit government agency. All employees, including doctors, are on salary, and decisions about care have no impact on any of their incomes. You have a strictly limited budget and you are told that you must limit expense for futile care at the end of life. Futile care is that given for patients for whom there is no hope that any intervention will change the outcome. Where do you draw the line?

Everyone on the committee agrees that Patient A deserves full-scale care. Patient B would probably garner about as many votes. Patients C and D are in an iffy zone; the committee is evenly split. E, F, and G are clearly futile and money spent on their care seems better spent elsewhere. They get no votes.

The Socialdom doctor who informs the family feels confident because it is not his decision, his financial concerns have not created any conflict, and it is for the public good. The family will likely respect the authority and the neutral nature of the decision and accept it.

Let us return to the United States. Now, if you can tolerate the thought, imagine first that each patient is your child, your spouse, or your parent, as would be appropriate to your situation, and then imagine yourself as each patient. Where would you draw the line for your loved one? Where for yourself? Does the cost matter to you in these personal choices? Each of us would draw a line at the level that fits our personal philosophy, needs, and beliefs. In actual practice today, the decision would not be yours to make.

Let us now imagine that the decision for each patient is in the hands of a large for-profit hospital corporation and its managed care insurance branch. Where do you think they would draw the divide as to which patient to fund and which to let die?

For many of us, prolonging suffering artificially is inhumane and unjustified. For many others, such as a wife who could not bring herself to authorize stopping her husband's life support, there are many reasons they would choose to continue care. If it were only a matter of preference, no one should want to intervene in a private decision. In reality, it is a matter of large sums of other people's money, as much as hundreds of thousands of dollars for a single ICU patient.

"Prognosis" means the forecast or the outcome of a disease. The last time you got soaked to the skin because the weather forecast was wrong when it predicted sunny skies should have taught you that a prognosis is only an estimate of probability. I have never said to a patient that someone will live a certain length of time or that a disease will go a certain way. That is a dishonest statement because we never *know* the future in any aspect of life, and medicine is no less so; we only calculate probability of what will be. I tell patients something like, "Most patients with this disease at this stage survive only a few months, but there is no way to know what will happen to you. You may want to be prepared in case you have that little time, but we can only wait and see how it will actually go." (I might note that the written word is much stiffer and harsher than what I would actually say in a real situation.)

One of my class's favorite teachers in medical school was a young instructor who was reportedly one of the most brilliant students to have graduated from the school, which if true, put him in remarkably august company. We were told the following story.

While performing an autopsy, his knife slipped and he was cut and infected with toxoplasmosis. Usually not serious, his case was said to have been so severe that he lapsed into a prolonged coma. The attending doctors despaired of his recovery and were going to end life support when, the story went, his friend, a fellow resident, told them they would do that only over his dead body. The teacher did eventually recover and spent the next years teaching, though there were some residual neurological deficits and he eventually succumbed to late complications. He was a terrific person and the extra years his friend won for him were well worth any expense.

Unfortunately, few people in what appears to be irreversible coma recover, and when they do, many are severely limited. Enough do survive, however, that when family members say that they have not given up hope, that they want to give more time for a miracle to occur, none of us can be sure that their hope is not justified.

This poses another dilemma. Do we continue extremely expensive life support for all to give the very few who defy the odds a chance to do so? If we do that, and if we have limited resources, how many patients will thus be deprived of care that is more likely to help?

We must decide how much "futile" care we are willing to pay for. If decisions must be made by someone other than the patient or the patient's designated representative, then who should make the decision?

THE SLIPPERY SLOPE

Let us accept that our limited resources have to be rationed *somehow* and that we must draw the line *somewhere*. How can we make the point of division acceptable to most people? Removing financial incentive is the first step. When decisions involve a conflict between what is right for the patient or for society and what is advantageous for the one making the decision, trust quickly evaporates. Trust is essential to authority that is based on moral integrity rather than brute physical power. If we trust our police, we will obey their directives. If we do not trust them, they will need their guns to enforce compliance with their orders. Trust requires moral integrity, unambiguous purpose, and convincing reason.

If you are the officer of a managed care corporation, your responsibility is to the shareholders of your corporation and your decisions affect the value of your stock options. Can your decisions be fully trusted? Obviously not, as few saints sit on boards of directors. You enforce your decision not by moral authority but by the power you wield. You have a contract signed by the patient, you are a billion-dollar corporation, and laws and legal precedents do not currently effectively limit your power.

"She is an old lady in the ICU and her case is hopeless, why waste money on her?" may evolve to, "She is an old lady. Maybe she is not hopeless, but why waste money on her?" Our executive begins to wonder why he should waste money on some homebound old man. His life may not seem very worthwhile to an ambitious executive looking to improve profits or to the lower-level employee who has to comply with company policy. Suppose that homebound man is your father . . . or you.

Rationalizations beget more rationalizations. Those inconvenient old people. Those retarded kids. Those . . . Should doctors have the power to end life? Should insurance executives or government bureaucrats have that power? Should families and patients be able to command extremely high-cost care? Should they have the right to high-cost care when it is futile? Where do we draw the line? How do we keep from sliding the line further and further down the slippery slope once we decide that someone other than the patient or the family can draw the line?

It is so much harder to know where to draw the line when those in power are not evil but they are not family, they may be well intentioned but concerned more for society than for the patient, or they may be influenced by their own financial incentives. These are not issues peculiar to managed care. These confront us under any payment system, and have since technology created the choices.

Remember that it may be you or your loved one in that bed. You may not want extraordinary care, preferring to go peacefully rather than delay the inevitable at a high cost in pain and suffering. Or, you may so ache at the thought of losing your loved one that you treasure every extra moment you can gain. What is right for you and your family may be judged differently by others.

HOW MUCH SHOULD DOCTORS EARN?

In a free-market system like America's, doctors should earn as much as they want and the market will bear. In terms of what is "right," however, doctors should earn as much as they want, within reason—but that should apply to every American in every occupation. To make the issue even more complex, who judges what is reasonable?

Discussing doctors' income is a thankless task. The concerted anti-doctor tone of the media over the past ten years has poisoned the reputation of the medical profession. The field has brought some of it on itself, but the vast majority of good doctors are smeared by the indiscriminate criticism of doctors as if all 750,000 were one person. The public's perception is that all doctors are rich and drive Mercedes. Personally, I wish it were true. I would be happy to have all the money that I am supposed to have.

Most doctors earn a good to very good living, but they do so more by the long hours they work than by the amount they are paid. Some doctors earn huge incomes because they have a unique skill or because they are among a small group whose field is unusually lucrative, such as neurosurgery or plastic surgery.

Suppose we say doctors' incomes should be limited to only $80,000 per year. Since they would not have to see as many patients, they could spend more time with each individual. In the world of managed care and most clinics, doctors are forced to see a high volume under threat of losing a contract or being fired, regardless of how much they earn. Thus, reducing income does not mean that time with patients will improve.

The most recent claim is that the average doctor makes in private practice $199,000.[9] That is a very misleading figure. If it were true, limiting income to $80,000 would entail a drop of 60 percent in income! Who among us could sustain such a dramatic loss?

Self-employed physicians have no job benefits to sustain them in difficult times. No employer pays for health insurance, life insurance, disability insurance, unemployment insurance, or malpractice insurance. Health, life, and disability insurance alone can cost $30,000.

The article says that the average internist earns $143,900. Even that is high because it lumps together doctors who simply spend time with patients and perform very few procedures and those doctors who have higher incomes from procedures, in-house laboratories, X-ray facilities, and the rest. These figures are from self-reported surveys by the AMA. I strongly suspect that they are skewed upward because the more successful doctors are the ones most likely to want to share their good fortune and the more mundane earners would have little interest in bothering with a survey.

People who can get through medical school might actually have done better in potentially more lucrative fields such as law or investment banking. One study compared the return on investment in time, tuition, and delayed income earning to be an investment banker versus two medical specialties, prior to managed care. A gastroenterologist then would have done a little better than the average investment banker, but a rheumatologist much worse. I am sure that the same study today under managed care would show the banker far outstripping either specialist.

I know by my own accurate but unofficial interviews that these income estimates are much too high for internists. The surgical and other procedural specialties may be a little closer to the real figures, but I am sure that they are skewed. However, suppose we accept the figure of $199,000 as accurate for purposes of discussion. The average work week for a doctor used to be sixty hours per week, but under the new economics, hours are even longer, so the average is now probably seventy hours per week.

Seventy hours per week for fifty weeks (we will give the doctor two weeks off) is 3,500 hours per year. Remember that this does not include reading the medical journals and books essential to remaining current in medical knowledge and skills. A salary of $199,000 divided by 3,500 hours is $57 per hour. In New York, the plumber who fixes the doctor's sink in his office charges $70 per hour or more. The repairman who comes to fix the broken $20 cable on the ECG machine bills his time at $125 per hour, minimum one hour, with an additional one hour billed for travel time even if he comes from next door. If the doctor needs a lawyer because the plumber flooded his office and destroyed half his practice, the lawyer charges $250 per hour. Prices in New York are higher than in most other parts of the country, but where the prices are lower, so are the incomes.

Those doctors who earn $100,000 for a seventy-hour week and have to pay $30,000 for the higher costs incurred by being self-employed and paying off educational loans, earn only $20 per hour.

Most doctors earn good incomes only because they work such long hours. Their hourly rate is quite reasonable compared to what we pay others in society, some of whose contributions are much less important than *saving your life.*

Now let us add in other factors to consider. A doctor has to remain in school until age twenty-six, not only earning nothing, but also running up an average debt of $150,000. The doctor then does housestaff training that can run from age twenty-six to as old as thirty-five, meanwhile working eighty to one hundred hours per week at salaries usually well below $30,000, and probably incurring even more debt.

Once the doctor can finally begin practice, the overhead to run an office and malpractice insurance must be paid even if there is not a single patient yet in the office. Malpractice insurance alone can cost more than $100,000 per year, depending on specialty and location. Because of managed care, few doctors today can open a solo practice (one doctor alone). Those remaining in solo practice are fading fast.

Most doctors today have seen sharp drops in their income. Some specialties and some individual doctors continue to make very high incomes, but they are probably a small minority, as best I can determine.

Some doctors are prospering more than ever under managed care because, if you play the game, you can share in the riches, though only those small leftovers dribbled down by the real winners, the executives and investors. Medical directors of managed care companies earn good incomes, especially if the doctor cooperates in denying a lot of care.

The primary doctors who are the alleged heroes of managed care do not make large salaries unless they fully participate in the managed care way. They work extraordinarily long, hard hours to maintain that income, at the heavy expense of stress, high risk, loss of personal life, and time stolen from their families.

Many doctors pay a very high price for this costly dedication.

Divorce, substance abuse, and suicide are more common among doctors. Their families also suffer as children grow up semiparentless. Spouses left at home pay their own dues in loneliness and isolation.

Most physicians chose medicine as a career because they prize independence and autonomy; desire to help others; are fascinated with the scientific wonder of life; and desire to earn a good living, respect, and stature in the community. No doctor I know entered medicine for what is experienced today: denying patients care, running patients through an assembly line, having little or no autonomy and independence, having time frittered away by mindless bureaucracy, struggling with the daily assaults to ethical standards, realizing that they are suffering all this to make profits for some distant businessperson whose only purpose is to make money. Do we really want to demoralize and abuse the very people who tend to us when we are ill, who struggle to convince us to live healthier lives, who have invested their lives in helping others?

Most doctors in my experience have a very strong sense of duty. They will persist in doing their best even under such an abusive system, but how long can that last? The men and women we call doctors and nurses are people just like you. They have families, needs, and feelings.

From my interviews with a large number of doctors and from my extensive research, I can report that the morale of the medical profession is astonishingly low. Even the staid medical literature is replete with articles expressing outrage, depression, and misery. Senior physicians are retiring from practice rather than submit to managed care. Their experience is an invaluable asset in medicine. How tragic if we should lose this treasured pool of wisdom. And most doctors I have interviewed tell me that they strongly advise young people not to choose medicine as a career because of managed care and Medicare.

While I believe the majority of doctors are very unhappy under managed care, there are some who are still satisfied: Those who are participating enthusiastically in managed care are enjoying the profits.

Some doctors' practices have so far been able to eschew managed care and yet retrain enough loyal followers to prosper. Large groups may create an *esprit de corps* that makes it easier for members to accept the restrictions and the ethical conflicts. Physicians in widespread networks may still retain a sense of the nonprofit collegiality that the network has incubated over the years. Large capitation groups may be caught up in the initial siren call of potential profits. Despite these exceptions, from my interviews and my literature research, I believe that most doctors do not feel anything but frustration and disgust.

I fear that we have not yet even begun to see the full repercussions of this crisis of spirit. Medicine is a profession that succeeds only by full and enthusiastic pursuit. Today, however, I often see patients who are refugees from managed care. A number of them are hurt by the recent change they have experienced with doctors they have seen for years and with whom they had felt very close. Now those same doctors are hard to see, and when appointments are obtained, the doctors are distant, sullen, and rushed, and spend five minutes with the patient, running to the next patient almost as they enter.

So, how much *should* doctors earn? The first answer again is that such a question is inappropriate. In the United States, we do not tell our citizens how much they can earn, how they live their lives, or how to think. If we did that, then the first question ought to be, how much can a managed care executive earn? Does it make sense for an executive to earn more than a neurosurgeon? Does it make sense for a doctor whose duty is to oppose or deny care to patients he or she has never seen to earn more than the physician administering the care? We are stepping onto another slippery slope when we begin to say that it is all right to regulate the income of this group or that, because, besides being unfair and un-American, it could spread to the next group and the next. Where would it stop?

Medicare and managed care *de facto* set doctors' incomes. Had the Clinton plan been enacted, it would have in effect controlled doctors' incomes. Single-payer and any form of national health insurance would do the same. We must decide if we are going to dictate to our doctors or if we are going to allow them the same freedom accorded all other Americans.

THE BEST COST AND QUALITY CONTROL

The best way to ensure quality care in medicine and to keep costs reasonable is by vigorously supporting and promoting research and by training good doctors. The best way to make good doctors is to begin with good people, see that they get a good education, create an atmosphere of decency and high ethical standards, provide them the time and the tools to offer good care, and allow them freedom to practice medicine with dignity and support. Good doctors practice good, cost-effective medicine.

As we noted previously, education and research are being seriously undermined by managed care and Medicare cutbacks in hospital profits in medical schools. We must decide whether we are going to directly fund the education and research that were previously subsidized indirectly by the teaching hospital "tax" (the practice of charging private pay and insurance customers more than the actual cost of procedures). All businesses charge more than their cost, but nonprofit hospitals used that profit to fund research, education, and care of the poor. Managed care used its buying power to force reductions in hospital profits.

This is a critical issue. Education and research are the future. Replacing retiring physicians with poorly trained people who are taught more about how to survive under managed care than how to be good doctors will destroy our health care system. Many infectious diseases have yet to be conquered. Many bacterial infections that were previously easily controlled are no longer always able to be cured because the bacteria are becoming resistant to antibiotics. There is still no drug that will kill viruses the way antibiotics kill bacteria. Diseases like HIV, Hantz virus, Lyme disease, and others are becoming more prevalent. We have won a lot of battles, but the war is far from over. Research is vital.

The baby boomers are the healthiest generation yet. Prior to them, most people thought of over-fifty as approaching old age and that they would decline from then on. The boomers are the first group to enter mid-life with the full expectation of continuing to be active and productive for the rest of their lives, possibly for another thirty or forty years. This means that they will be placing great demands on the medical system to keep them healthy, which can be met only by strong investment in research in every area.

In 1995, the United States spent $16.6 billion on medical research and over $52 billion on amusement and recreation services.[10] We all want to have fun, and there is no reason to deprive ourselves of it, but we also have to be healthy to enjoy it.

Of course, I cannot fail to note that the surest way to a healthy, productive, long life depends on the least expensive factors: proper nutrition, regular vigorous exercise, reasonable screening to detect disease early, remaining active and positive, forming strong social relationships, and learning to improve emotional control.

SPECIALISTS

In the early days of modern medicine, most doctors were general practitioners (GPs). They went into practice after one year of internship in a hospital. They took care of adults, children, and babies; they delivered babies; set fractures; gave B_{12} shots (as a tonic, whether needed or not); cleaned wax from ears; and even did routine surgeries. (The closest to this today are specialists called family practitioners, but they serve a full residency after internship.)

As medicine progressed, the knowledge needed in each area exploded beyond the ability of any one person to master, so specialization began to be an important component of medical care. As the complexity and wealth of knowledge continued to increase, subspecialties developed.

It is impossible today for any physician to know all of medicine, or even all of a specialty or even a subspecialty. For example, endocrinology is a subspecialty of the specialty known as internal medicine. Endocrinology studies diseases of the glands that excrete hormones. Some endocrinologists see all kinds of patients in their subspecialty, but many concentrate on and only see patients with disease of only one gland, such as diabetes, thyroid disease, or pituitary disease. Specialists are an invaluable tool for the care of patients. I believe that every patient should have a general doctor (I vote for the internist, for obvious reasons, but also because I feel we have the most intensive training in the diseases of adults) who takes care of them as a whole person and coordinates all of their care. The patient's doctor* can call in specialists as needed.

I use specialists liberally and frequently. If someone else knows about an aspect of the patient's problem better than I do, I want my patient to have the most knowledgeable care possible. But I do not turn the patient over to the specialist. Just the opposite is true: I continue to be the patient's doctor, I work with the consultants and follow the patient closely, making sure everything is coordinated and that the patient understands all that is being done and why. The patient needs a doctor who will fully coordinate everything that happens to the patient. As I said before, we must not take care of the patient's organs with a different specialist working on each one. We must take care of the patient as a whole person who may have dysfunction in one area or another.

The patient should get the finest care available. Physicians should know where they are fully able to handle a problem and where additional input is needed. I tell patients that three of the most important

---

*"Primary doctor" used to be an acceptable term, but today it so closely associated with managed care that I am avoiding it to prevent confusion.

words in medicine are "I don't know." If you sense that your doctor does not know those words, watch out—no doctor knows everything and the best doctors know the boundaries of their knowledge.

The issue for the cost watchers is whether we should pay for specialist care. Specialists' fees are sometimes higher, as their unique skills might command, but we should expect to pay for what we get if they are. It is said by managed care advocates that specialists order more tests and spend more to justify their existence. That is absurd. Good doctors order what the patient needs. The whole point of using specialists is that they have training in the use of the more sophisticated diagnostic tools available to their specialty. Those advanced techniques pay off in better care, which is always more cost effective than poor care.

Some doctors have developed special skills that no one else can duplicate. Dr. Fred Epstein is a famous example. His special skill relates to tumors in children and some adults that invade the spinal cord and move up to the brain. These tumors twist in and around the cord in a way that would make them seemingly impossible to remove without badly damaging the normal tissue. Somehow, Epstein succeeds where no other doctor does. He has done well over five hundred of these procedures, and he has frequently done them for free when patients in need cannot afford them.

In 1995, a thirty-year-old woman who had been struggling with such a tumor for fifteen years was getting worse despite all treatment. She was told by her HMO neurosurgeon that she needed the operation and that only Epstein could do it. According to an article in the *New York Post*, her HMO, HIP Health Plan of New Jersey, refused to authorize Epstein to do it.[11] Epstein then offered to perform the surgery free, foregoing his usual $12,000 fee. The HMO refused to pay the hospital bill unless the operation was done by a neurosurgeon in their network. That surgeon had *never* done this incredibly difficult procedure. The HMO was quoted as saying that the difference between the two surgeons was "splitting hairs."

Practice makes a difference. There have been many studies that show unequivocally that experience in any procedure makes a huge difference in success and safety. To send a patient to a doctor totally inexperienced in one of the most difficult procedures in neurosurgery is an egregious affront to decency. If the newspaper account is accurate (the series was edited by a Pulitzer Prize–winning journalist), this illustrates just how bad the system can be.

Today, doctors report significant difficulty in referring to specialists under managed care.[12] Thus, the issue is, do we want to have access to the best care or do we want such access limited, as is allegedly necessary to save money?

LONG TERM OR SHORT TERM?

One reason that people have trouble losing weight is that the donut in front of them is right now, but the heart attack such fatty foods might cause is some vague possibility that seems far in the future. If you put money into a savings fund, you do with a little less now for the hope of some compounded nest egg for the future. Executives often have to choose between a short-term action of little value that will boost the value of their stock for a short while versus reducing their earnings reports to invest in growth that will come long after they are retired. Their stock options will only benefit from the short-term action.

Managed care is concerned only with short-term results. It needs to show short-term high returns for those who invest or they will sell their stock and invest elsewhere. There is a high turnover rate among their customers.[13] Employers change plans often and employees can choose different plans among the choices offered. Why should managed care companies invest in the care of people they think may not be with them long? There is a steady consolidation in the managed care industry, so executives never know if *they* will be there tomorrow.

In contrast, everything about good health care is investing for the future. I tell my patients that the maximum human lifespan (as of now) is 120 years, as I noted before, and that while I take care of any immediate problems, I am just as interested or more so in how they do for the rest of their lives. It obviously costs more in the short run, though not much more, to take care of the future as well as the present, but the payoff for society is rich in value and less in cost in the end. Unless one cares only about short-term gain, the best investment is obviously the one for the fullest, longest life people can reasonably attain.

Even in the short run, better care, while sometimes more expensive at first, is always cheaper in the end, because good results cost less than bad ones. A poor outcome for the patient who wanted to see Fred Epstein would cost much more in a prolonged hospitalization, rehabilitation costs, and long-term care.

POOR DISTRIBUTION OF HEALTH CARE

Farmers feed us, but if they get sick or injured, who is there to help? There are far fewer doctors in rural areas. How many doctors choose to practice in inner cities? To whom do Native Americans, the impoverished ones who do not have oil wells and casinos, turn when they need medical care? Our infant death rate is higher than it should be, primarily because of poverty; lack of inner city health care; poor, young, unwed parents; drug use; and HIV. Compounding these causes is the lack of medical care for these mothers and their babies.

Most of the care for the inner cities and other poor neighborhoods falls to the few municipal hospitals in these areas. Overloaded and underfunded, they have to struggle to provide even minimal care. There is no easy solution to this problem. It takes unusually dedicated people to choose to practice in the areas of greatest need but least attractiveness. There are those very dedicated few who do, but nowhere near enough. We must decide if we are willing to spend the extra funds to provide enough monetary compensation to balance the disadvantages to doctors who can choose to practice anywhere.

The disastrous effects of managed care on some doctors have pushed them to answer the calls of smaller communities, but not enough. We need to develop innovative ways of delivering care to underserved areas. In rural areas, we could set up central facilities and send out doctors by helicopter to make rounds over broad areas, for example. There has been increasing use of airplanes and helicopters to reach patients in isolated areas and bring them to a facility for emergency or other special care not available locally.

Technology may solve some of the problem. Telemedicine, providing medical consultation and care over video and computer hookups, is developing some exciting new possibilities. The capability exists to televise patients, even operations, to distant consultants who supervise the care almost as if they were in the same room. Remote robotics may allow the consultant to examine patients from a distance. It is said that the robots will eventually be able to even transmit skin sensory information like texture and temperature and perhaps even odor. Surgeons will be able to operate on a distant patient by remote control of robotic arms. Already consultants can review digitized X-rays and EKGs in real time and give immediate feedback to the local doctor.

This of course is not the same as meeting face to face, and distant video connections do not duplicate a family doctor in your community whom you know and can see when needed. One challenge, as with any use of computers and electronic communication, is to preserve privacy.

HOW MUCH SHOULD WE EXPECT?

Remember C. Everett Koop's statement that the greediest participants in health care are the patients? We all want the best for ourselves and our families. Well, of course we do. What Dr. Koop meant was that many of us have *excessive* expectations regarding what our current health care is capable of. Some of us want more than we need; others expect medicine to solve problems beyond its current capabilities.

This is a different issue than rationing. Rationing is the imposition of limits on individuals by society to better distribute limited resources for the public good. What we are now discussing is how individuals decide how they will use their own resources. If something is free, the natural tendency is to want as much as you can get.

If there is a cost to something, then we each make our own decision as to how much we are willing to spend for that service. Before health insurance, it was relatively simple—people purchased as much health care as they needed and could afford. Health insurance became necessary when costs became too high for too many people, but it started the process of separating service from its direct cost. Once health insurance buffered people from most of the cost, utilization soared. Doctors pursued their natural course to provide the best they could for patients. The fact that nonrestraint was also beneficial to the doctor was an inflationary factor to some degree, but one held in check by the natural inclination of a good doctor to do no more than was necessary.

When society broke the covenant with physicians, things changed. (The covenant was that doctors gave their all for their patients in return for respect, stature in the community, and a good living.) As the tide turned and physicians became the object of society's scorn in the battle for control of health care dollars—a very one-sided battle that most doctors did not even realize was going on—doctors were put on the defensive and their judgment was questioned mercilessly.

I have said that physicians' responsibility is not to total society health care costs. I have spent this entire book explaining why neither government nor profit-minded businesspeople should make these decisions. Then who should?

The answer is easy: *You* should. You, the patient, should decide how much of your money is spent on health care. If you are spending your *own* money, you will spend only what you absolutely need, so that you have some left over to pay for other wants and needs. Corporations demanded managed care to reduce their own costs, but nothing in managed care permits individuals to have a say in how their premium dollars are spent for the patients' own, unique needs.

How do we change the system so patients begin to self-regulate their health care utilization? We will discuss that in the last chapter.

WHAT CAUSES THE MOST HEALTH CARE COSTS?

You cause the most health care costs—if you smoke, overeat, drink excessively, use drugs, shoot guns at people, behave recklessly by not wearing a seatbelt, or put your life at risk in the careless pursuit of thrills. Shall we regulate all these things out of existence? Even if we could, which is doubtful, do we want to? Do we want a country that tells people how to live? As a society we have amply indicated that we do not. Then how about all the people who live their lives without these dangerous actions? Should they have to subsidize the expensive care of those who indulge?

There are no easy answers to the questions of whether it is government's job to protect people from themselves or whether one should pay for another's indulgence, or where to draw the line if we did. These are societal questions, not medical ones. The medical answer is easy—do not indulge. The societal question has as many answers as there are people.

It is much easier to support efforts to protect nonusers from ancillary effects of users' habits: Government should do all in its power to keep people from drinking and driving. No one should have to involuntarily breathe in smoke. Drug users should be prevented from stealing to pay for their habit, if drugs continue to be illegal. If IV drug users contract HIV or tuberculosis, as so many do, great effort should be made to prevent transmission to unsuspecting partners or to the public.

My own personal calculation, based on thirty years of observation and study, is that most likely tobacco accounts for or contributes to at least one-third of all health care costs, alcohol and drugs probably for another quarter, and improper nutrition and lack of exercise for another third. This would leave less than 10 percent due solely to other causes.

Do we want to pay such a high price for the freedom to pollute ourselves? My own choice for myself is to use no tobacco, alcohol, or drugs; to eat as healthily as I can; and to exercise regularly. I follow the advice I give my patients, but notice that I said advice that I *give*. Giving advice and imposing choices are two different things. Society has been ambivalent. We allow smoking and ban heroin, even though the former is a thousand times more dangerous than the latter.* We watch drunk drivers slaughter our children and families in tens of thousands of collisions. So far we have had little success in curbing drunk driving. We write about healthy food but use all the incredible power of advertising to sell people the unhealthiest foods possible. And so it goes.

Americans value their freedom of choice very highly. (Perhaps we should rise *en masse* against managed care, which steals choice from us as few businesses do.) We can only educate people as to the consequences of their choices and hope for the best. However, we must not delude ourselves; we will continue to have high health care costs as long as we continue to pollute and endanger ourselves.

ALTERNATIVE MEDICINE

Many factors are fueling the rise of alternative medicine. For some it seems more attuned to their own beliefs and lifestyles. For some, it is the alternative of last hope when traditional treatments fail. Some turn to alternative care when, under managed care, their doctors have no time for them. Many people are enticed by the promises of miraculous effects from "natural" treatments.

Alternative care is risky, as it is untested and unproven. Mainstream medicine has risks as well. Anytime you intervene with a treatment, no matter what, there is always a risk. The difference is in the attempts made to eliminate as much risk and uncertainty as possible before introducing a new treatment into general use. I would vote for the same strict regulation of alternative care as is applied to mainstream medicine. I would be overjoyed if the many claims for alternative treatments were validated, and I would enthusiastically offer them to my patients if their therapeutic value were scientifically verified.

The first three words in medicine are "Do no harm!" It is essential for every doctor to know, as well as possible, the risk of any treatment and whether it is likely to help. This is impossible with alternative care,

---

*Pure heroin, used in correct dosage with sterile technique, is amazingly safe physically. It *is* addicting and *can* seriously impair performance and enjoyment of life, so it is certainly not good for you.

whose treatments are inadequately tested for efficacy or safety. For example, we in the United States strictly regulate the use of prescription drugs. While some have been converted to over-the-counter forms, which is risky at best, most remain available to people only by a doctor's prescription. You cannot go to the drugstore and buy an antibiotic of your choice without a prescription. In most other countries, this is not the case. In some, only narcotics require prescriptions. If you wish, you can treat yourself with most medications without ever seeing a doctor.

Misuse of medications is very hazardous. Even physicians have to work very hard to make sure we use them correctly and safely—what chance does a layperson have with no medical training? The information available to the public from books, magazines, broadcasting, the Internet, and your local pharmacists (when they give advice how to treat rather than on how to use a drug) is unreliable. Drug companies are now marketing prescription drugs directly to consumers in the hope that we will demand these products from our doctors. Can you imagine what it would be like if they could try to convince you to use their drugs without having to see a doctor? Perhaps you will hear a clever jingle, like, "Cure-All tastes good, like an anticancer drug should!" Even proper information is meaningless out of the context of full training in medicine. In addition, you cannot be objective about yourself. Even doctors should see other doctors for their own health care.

If you harm yourself or make yourself worse by self-diagnosis and treatment, who pays to treat the resulting medical problems? Should other people carry higher premiums to pay for your choice? For instance, misuse of antibiotics harms us all. We already face a newly reinvigorated army of microbes which have found ways to defeat our most powerful drugs. Inappropriate or incorrect use of antibiotics helps the microbes to develop resistance. Self-treatment is a poor practice and a potentially dangerous one, but should you have the right to make that choice for yourself?

In effect, alternative medicine is the same as self-treatment of any other kind. What makes it more difficult is that its claims of efficacy, safety, and usefulness are unsubstantiated in any valid, reproducible way. There is no way to support these claims through independent means. Society must decide whether freer choice of treatment, without adequate information on which to base such a choice, is worth the hazards.

POVERTY

No discussion of health care costs can be complete without discussing poverty and homelessness.

That there are children in America who go hungry or who live on the street is simply unacceptable and sickening. As the lucky upper echelons wallow joyfully in the continuing strong economy, the poor and homeless are the forgotten. Somehow, they were a big story in the 1980s and now they do not exist.

Well, they are still out there, shivering, stomachs in pain from hunger, some as badly off as those we occasionally see in stories on poor developing countries. Can't each of us spare a little for them? So much of some charitable contributions go to those raising the funds or are wasted by inefficiency, couldn't we find simple ways to help our less fortunate neighbors directly?

There were 36.4 million Americans below the poverty level in 1995 compared to 25.9 million in 1975. They are comprised of every ethnic group, including more than half Caucasian, so poverty is an equal opportunity nonemployer. We do not know how many homeless there are. The 1990 census estimated that there were more than 228,621 homeless people, over 50 percent of whom were in families with children.[14]

Poverty and malnutrition are major causes of high health care costs, because we do eventually take care of them, only we wait until they are so far advanced that they cost much more. A bowl of soup is a lot cheaper than a hospital bed and intravenous antibiotics. A decent home and a job are a lot less expensive than advanced cancer.

DO WE PAY EQUALLY OR ACCORDING TO NEED?

There are two ways to set insurance premiums. In community rated plans everyone pays the same regardless of medical condition or risk. The total cost of providing care plus administrative cost and profit is divided by the number of people covered. A twenty-five-year-old would pay the same as an ill seventy-year-old smoker. Then there is underwriting in which experts analyze the risk factors, including age, gender, health history, and things like blood pressure, cholesterol, and smoking for each applicant, and then adjust the premium to match the risk. The ill seventy-year-old smoker would pay much more than the healthy twenty-five-year-old would. This is called experience-rating in insurance terms.

Community rating at first favors the higher-risk person and increases the premium of those at a low risk. However, the healthy may choose to drop out of the insurance pool, which reduces the number of people available to divide the premium among. The premium may then become very high for the remaining, higher-risk people if too many healthy people drop out.

If everyone *had* to have insurance so that there were no drop-outs, then the question remains: Should the healthy members subsidize the cost for the unhealthy members? Of course, any low-risk person could suddenly switch sides and become an unhealthy if he does not wear a seatbelt or if he eats or smokes himself into an illness or contracts some other disease.

We may spend a huge amount of money for life insurance which we dearly hope we will never use, or at least not for a very expensively long time. Why waste money? Because we want our families to be protected just *in case!* That is what insurance is for: in case. None of us is safe.

Life insurance is always underwritten, at least by age and most often also by health and habits. Should we do the same for health insurance? Should we all pay the same to help the sick, the old, and the weak, or should we charge them more to keep rates down for the youngsters whose incomes are usually lower and need to get a good start? The decisions never seem to end.

WHOSE LIFE IS IT?

Just how responsible for ourselves are we? If we choose to smoke, drink, overeat, save money by not buying insurance, or drive without a seatbelt, who takes care of us if we pay the likely price for risky behavior and become ill and need care? If I spend thousands of dollars per year on health insurance and you merrily save that money to spend on other things, is it my responsibility to pay for your care if you get sick?

If you smoke and I drink, are we equally risking ourselves? It is pretty close (smoking wins by far but alcohol tries hard as number two). If you smoke and I do not wear a seatbelt, are they equal? How about if you smoke and I climb a mountain? Life is to live; there is no way to compare risky sports to smoking.

These are vital questions when we come to who pays what. Should we draw a line? If so, where? No one could dispute that use of tobacco and excessive alcohol are extremely high risk activities and not very productive. Yet there are smokers and drinkers who think that it is a great way to live and that no one should question their choices in a free country. Some—a very few—are even lucky enough to survive without adverse effects. They would say that none of us is perfect and that we all have some bad habits.

How do we rate overeating? That kills almost as many people as smoking, but we all *have* to eat and it can be difficult to do it right in industrialized, urban cultures. Should we be penalized if we get one of the many weight/fat-related diseases? What about people who eat no vegetables? Where do we draw the line between personal choice and imposing our problems unfairly on others?

Should the government act as a surrogate parent to force us all to control our habits to reduce health care costs, or are we to remain proud and independent and free to damage ourselves as much as we want?

HOW DO WE PAY FOR EXPENSIVE PROCEDURES THAT ARE PREVENTIVE OR CONSIDERED BY SOME TO BE UNPROVEN?

George J. Annas, a lawyer who has written extensively on legal issues in medicine, has addressed some of the challenging issues raised by genetic diseases.[15] He writes of a woman whose mother and aunt had both died of ovarian cancer, giving her and her sisters a 50 percent chance of contracting the same disease (women with no family history have only a 1.5 percent risk). Ovarian cancer is very difficult to detect early enough to cure (as described in the story of beloved comedienne Gilda Radner's struggle with ovarian cancer, *Gilda's Disease*).[16] The woman's doctor recommended prophylactic (preventive) removal of her uterus and ovaries. The insurance company refused to pay for it. It eventually went to the Nebraska Supreme Court, which ruled in the patient's favor.

We will be facing increasingly difficult questions with our new ability to detect genes that pose a risk. There are no right answers and society will have to decide how to deal with all the implications of emerging genetic knowledge.

What shall we do about so-called experimental treatments, such as bone marrow transplants? One person's experiment is another's hope for recovery. I think these decisions are easily made. If there were no established successful treatments for serious or life-threatening diseases, most people would want to try a procedure that at least had a chance of working even if it were not yet fully proven. That then raises a new quandary—does "experimental" include unproven or discredited remedies, such as the alternative treatment laetrile, claimed to be a cancer cure? The National Cancer Institute studied laetrile and showed that it is worthless, but I am sure there are still those who believe in it. A patient might say he had incurable cancer and wanted to try this as a last resort. If we pay for a bone marrow transplant, why not laetrile? As a specialist in internal medicine, I know that bone marrow transplants may well help many people, even if conclusive studies are still in progress, because I understand its science, use, and results in the context of my overall knowledge, but that does not resolve the issue for those who favor laetrile.

We need to establish mechanisms to resolve these kinds of questions as well as how to handle the costs that result. I believe strongly that these decisions must be made independent of the profit considerations inherent in managed care.

WHO DECIDES HOW MUCH CARE YOU RECEIVE?

I believe *you* should decide how much care you receive. We cannot afford to pay for all the care that everyone *wants*, but we must be able to afford to pay for all the care that each person *needs*. (By this I mean that no one should suffer unnecessary harm from lack of access to good medical care. Many people, when they are not spending their own money, want as much care as they can get, regardless of need or cost. When you spend your own money, you are far more likely to spend it as reasonably as you know how.)

Today, with the exception of the few remaining people who have traditional indemnity insurance or who are rich enough to pay all their costs themselves, how much care you get is decided for you by either managed care or the government.

How do we resolve this? I believe it is much simpler than it seems. In the final chapter I will propose a new system that I believe will accomplish the goals of restoring your right to decide your own health care for nearly every need, preserve your privacy and autonomy far more than under managed care and government programs, and put a sensible brake on runaway health costs.

TAXES AND UNCOMPENSATED CARE

The National Center for Policy Analysis (NCPA), a nonprofit research group, has done an interesting analysis of the tax implications of employee health benefits, such as health insurance, dental plans and the like, using 1995 as an example.[17] If an employee is paid $40,000 per year in salary, that amount is taxable, but if the employee receives $35,000 in salary and $5,000 in health care benefits, the $5,000 is not taxable. If the individual's total tax burden is, say, 25 percent, then the employee's taxes on benefits worth $5,000 is $1,250 less than if the compensation were pure salary. The national annual cost of the tax effects of health benefits given to employees as benefits instead of taxable wages amounts to *$86 billion* per year for the federal government and *$10 billion* for state governments.

Employers save on taxes by deducting the cost of health benefits for their employees. Those who buy their own insurance, such as self-employed people, are worse off. They pay for their own insurance with *after*-tax dollars, which is more expensive, and they can deduct health expenses only if they itemize deductions on their personal tax filings, and only those expenses that exceed 7.5 percent of adjusted gross income. While that is not a full deduction, it still provides at least some tax deduction that is not available to uninsured people, who are the worst off at tax time because they have nothing to deduct. On average, the increase in taxes for the uninsured amounts to $450 per year for the bottom fifth in income distribution and $1,780 per year for the top fifth, or $1,018 on average. Collectively, uninsured people pay *$19 billion* more in federal and state taxes than do people of similar income who receive the tax break.

What do uninsured people cost when they receive health care from hospitals, doctors, and other sources for which they cannot pay? Are they "freeloading?" There are two kinds of uncompensated care. The first is when people are uninsured and cannot pay the full cost of their care, nevertheless receive unpaid-for care from doctors, clinics, and hospitals. The Congressional Budget Office, NAPA reports, estimates this at about $27.6 billion for 1995. That sounds like the uninsured are costing everyone else $8.6 billion (the difference between the cost of their uncompensated care, $27.6 billion, and the higher taxes they pay compared to insured people, $19 billion). However, NAPA notes that the Congressional Budget Office has also estimated that there is a considerable amount of uncompensated care in Medicaid and Medicare. That is because those government programs require by law that hospitals, doctors, and others charge the program beneficiaries significantly lower fees than they do private patients. Thus, the amount that the care *would* have cost minus the amount Medicare and Medicaid actually spend is considered the amount of uncompensated care in those programs. In summary, of the total uncompensated care in the country, Medicare represented 33.0 percent, Medicaid, 42.6 percent and the uninsured only 24.3 percent, as shown in figure 12.1:

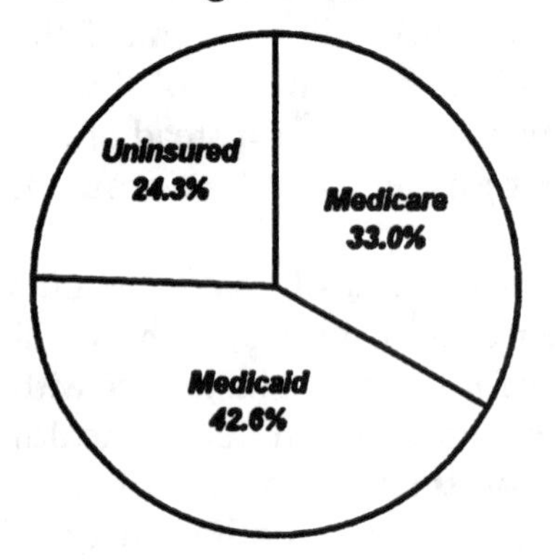

Fig. 12.1. Share of Uncompensated Care

As we have discussed at length in this book, the uninsured get inadequate care. I feel that in managed care, Medicare, and Medicaid underfunding of needed care has similar adverse effects.

HOW MUCH OF OUR RESOURCES SHOULD WE DEVOTE TO HEALTH CARE?

Currently we spend a little over 14 percent of GDP on health care in the United States. That is higher than any other country, but our needs and demands are higher also. Where we fail is in the abuses of managed care, in not providing care for everyone, and in providing inadequate care for those who need long-term assistance. To improve the care of the underserved, we will have to spend more money.

Whenever we say we must spend more, the answer immediately is that we will have to give up education, defense, or some other vital service. The immediate answer to health needs is always that we have "limited resources." After all, our total GDP is only *$7 trillion* per year.

The new health care system I recommend in the last chapter

should save billions by eliminating waste. Reducing excess administrative costs will not deprive anyone of care (in fact, it will improve it). This will finance new programs.

I can think of a few areas where we spend money that might be a little less important than education or health: Americans spent an astonishing *$586.5 billion* in 1996 on gambling, and even more each succeding year![18] That is half a trillion dollars. Does it make any sense for a child to be sleeping in a cardboard box while a celebrity loses $165,000 in one night in a casino? It is his money to do with as he wishes, but what has become of us? Is it really better to pay a basketball player $100 million while people go without food? Suppose he only made $90 million and the other $10 million was used to give care to needy infants? Would he be so discouraged that he would shoot fewer baskets? This is an obvious, easy target (and he is seven feet tall), but there are many people with salaries so high they make no sense.

Athletes are small potatoes compared to business folk. *Business Week* reported that the average chief executive officer compensation package in 1997 was $7.8 million.[19] These salaries were *not* related to performance, increased even when the companies they ran did poorly, and in some cases the salaries even contributed to putting their companies into the red. The leader last year was Sanford Weill of Travellers Corporation, who has just planned a merger with Citicorp that will make him even richer. Weill's compensation package in 1997 was $230,725,000! He is a brilliant financier who has created jobs and economic wealth, but if he made only $100,000,000, do you think he would feel it was not worth it and would have run his company less well?

The head of Cedant was listed as sitting on $832,972,000 in stock options before the company developed problems. The NBC evening news of May 12, 1998, reported a story of a three-year-old very bright cerebral palsy child who was benefiting from rehabilitation until Oxford HMO told the parents their coverage was used up (that does not happen easily in traditional indemnity insurance). How many disabled children could $832 million help?

If Bill Gates gave away *half* of his fortune, he would still be worth $25 *billion!* He says he will, some day.

The head of Oxford HMO allegedly ran the company into the ground and was finally removed. He was "punished" with a $9 million goodbye gift (some of which was at least held back in response to public outrage). How many denied critical medical procedures did Oxford have to impose on its customers to scrape that together?[20]

When you read earlier in this chapter that Dr. Fred Epstein charges

$12,000 for one operation, that may have seemed like a lot, but a stockbroker can earn that in a three-minute trade over the telephone. Epstein has spent a career developing a skill that perhaps no one else has, one that can save the lives of children and allow them to function. The operation takes as much as twenty hours of punishing physical and mental stress. Playing basketball is a lot easier. There are many basketball players, but only one Fred. Are our priorities in the right place?

I love dogs and animals and our dog is a valued member of our family. Yet I marvel that it can now cost more to take a dog to a veterinarian than managed care or Medicare will allow for a human to visit a doctor! What's the matter with us?

A friend once told me about a letter he had read in a newspaper. A doctor had written that he had just consulted a lawyer for some simple legal work. The lawyer told him that the fee was $185 per hour (which is very reasonable for New York City lawyers). He finished his business, paid the lawyer and then went back to his office. By chance, the first patient waiting for him was a lawyer. This lawyer's law firm had a capitated managed care contract which paid the doctor $145 for the entire year's care of that lawyer patient. The doctor asked, "What has society come to if we value one hour of a lawyer's time more than one *year* of a doctor's time?"

The list is endless. Today there is probably a greater concentration of wealth in fewer hands than at any time in American history, and maybe in world history.

I wish all those lucky folk well and I wish I were among them, but I frankly get upset when I hear that there is not enough money to help people in need.

If the wealthiest 2 percent of the people in this country gave just 10 percent of their wealth into a fund for the poor and the underserved, we could probably wipe out poverty. Ted Turner has shown how to do it: He has given away nearly half of his fortune, gifts totaling well over a billion dollars. So has George Soros. They deserve muchcredit. They still have a lot left, so they have proved that they could have their cake and give some of it away, too.

I would love to see my taxes go down and I agree that low taxes promote economic growth. Americans hate taxes, but the fact is we have the *lowest* tax burden of any developed country in the world.

Are these the proper priorities for us? Do we really want to shortchange our own care, ignore our least fortunate, neglect our aging parents and watch as people suffer needlessly, just so we can gamble, watch overpaid athletes, allow executives to gorge themselves, take better care of our pets than of ourselves, and spend small fortunes with lawyers for every transaction? It is time to face simple facts. Every one of us will age and as we age we will need health care. The money we save scrimping on health care now in order to gamble, indulge, or entertain ourselves will come back to haunt us when we need help.

An easy way to attack my ideas would be to exaggerate what I am saying. We do *not* have to give up our pleasures, nor would I want to. We do need to keep our priorities straight and to spend a *little* less—I cannot emphasize this enough, I mean a *little* less—on the unnecessary to ensure that we are prepared for the important needs.

This quandary—the temptation of current gratification versus preparation for longer-term benefit—is one of humankind's oldest struggles, for which I certainly do not pretend to have a solution. We cannot legislate or enforce a sensible balance, but perhaps if each of us encourages others, we might just influence behavior enough to make a difference.

Look at the price we have already paid for managed care, which snuck in on us because we did not want to spend so much on health care. Now we are spending more and getting less. The proposals I make in the last chapter would improve health care and still permit us a great life. Many of the recommendations would likely save so much money that we might well be able to finance much more than we do now without spending more.

We can revolutionize medical care by eliminating administrative waste, by kicking out those who extract your dollars for their own profit; by empowering people to make their own choices; by improving prevention and the quality of care; and by better utilizing technology. This would initially spare us tax increases and pay for health care for the uninsured and the homeless. Eventually, the aging of America will catch up with us. Furthermore, there will be unbelievable political resistance to the changes I have suggested, and we may just stay where we unhappily are. In either case, we may eventually face having to spend increasing amounts of our wealth on staying healthy enough to enjoy it. We will finally have to face up to our obligations to our fellow Americans who are less fortunate, the homeless and the poor. I personally would spend even as high as 19 or 20 percent of the GDP to improve health and to fight poverty, especially if it is spent efficiently in the ways that I have outlined. We have learned through sad experience that welfare programs and the like do not work. I believe the plan I outline in the last chapter would avoid most if not all of the pitfalls of government programs. Outside of health care, the solutions to poverty and homelessness are not to throw money at them, but to use productive approaches such as job creation, education, and home ownership to give pride and responsibility. If *you* look a homeless child in the eye or watch a mother dying of breast cancer or see a powerful man felled by crushing pain in his chest, the number of people who agree with me might grow by one. If each of us stops our daily whirlwind of activity and thinks for a while about what really counts in life, maybe my little army will swell to an irresistible tide.

I am not suggesting that we all become saints living monastic lives. We can enjoy our lives just as we do now but we could shift our priorities a *little* to gain a lot.

Health care decisions must be made by all of us. Most of us do not think about these issues, however. We are all so busy with what we do every day that we rarely spend time thinking about issues vital to our lives. Just look at how few of us vote.

Your health is your *most* important asset—think for a moment what else would matter as much if your health were gone.

In the final chapter, we will try to figure out how to resolve the conflicts in health care and how to get good care at a reasonable price. There are no perfect answers, but I think we can find a way far superior to what we have now.

As we ponder the hows, keep remembering the whys. Look in the mirror, look at your family, and think about your priorities. Do not wait until it is too late.

NOTES

1. Uwe Reinhardt, "Wanted—A Clearly Articulated Social Ethic for American Health Care," *Journal of the American Medical Association* 278 (November 5, 1997): 1446–47.

2. R. A. Epstein, D. Lindsay, J. Lally, and U. Reinhardt, "Letters," *Journal of the American Medical Association* 279 (March 11, 1998): 745–46.

3. Personal communication from Monroe Trout, M.D.

4. Paul T. Menzel, *Strong Medicine, the Ethical Rationing of Health Care* (New York: Oxford University Press, 1990).

5. Martin Strosberg et al., *Rationing America's Medical Care: The Oregon Plan and Beyond* (Washington, D.C.: The Brookings Institute, 1992); Thomas Bodenheimber, "The Oregon Health Plan—Lessons for the Nation," *New England Journal of Medicine* 337 (August 28, 1997; September 4, 1997): 651–55, 720–23; Barbara Alden Wilson, "Is the Oregon Health Plan Working?" *Unique Opportunities* (January 1996): 32–39.

6. Jerry A. Menikoff, "The Role of the Physician in Cost Control," *Ophthalmology Clinics of North America* 10, no. 2 (June 1997): 191–95; Menzel, *Strong Medicine.*

7. David A. Asch and Peter A. Ubel, "Sounding Board: Rationing by Any Other Name," *New England Journal of Medicine* 336 (June 5, 1997): 1668–71.

8. Ruth Macklin, *Mortal Choices* (Boston: Houghton Mifflin, 1987), 105–106; David J. Rothman, *Strangers at the Bedside* (New York: Basic Books, 1991), 223–46.

9. Peter T. Kilborn, "Doctors' Pay Regains Ground Despite the Effects of HMOs," *New York Times,* April 22, 1998, A1, A20.

10. John W. Wright, ed., *The New York Times 1998 Almanac* (New York: Penguin Group, 1997), pp. 328, 382.

11. Cathy Burke, "Dying Woman Denied Doc She Needs," in "What You Don't Know about HMOs Could Kill You," *New York Post,* September 21, 1995, 15.

12. Karen Scott Collins, Cathy Schoen, and Daniel R. Sandmon, "The Commonwealth Fund Survey of Physician Experiences with Managed Care," March 1997, The Commonwealth Fund, http://www.cmwf.org/health_care/physrug.html, pp. 12–13.

13. Ibid., p. 9.

14. Ronald J. Alsop, ed., *The Wall Street Journal Almanac 1998* (New York: Dow Jones Co., 1997), p. 271.

15. George J. Annas, "When Should Preventive Treatment Be Paid for by Health Insurance?" *New England Journal of Medicine* 331 (October 3, 1994): 1027–34.

16. M. Steven Piver, *Gilda's Disease* (Amherst, N.Y.: Prometheus Books, 1996).

17. National Center for Policy Analysis, "Are the Uninsured Freeloaders?" http://www.publicpolicy.org/~ncpa/ba/ba120.html, August 21, 1998.

18. Ronald J. Alsop, ed., *The Wall Street Journal Almanac 1998* (New York: Dow Jones Co., 1997), p. 935.

19. Jennifer Reingold, "Executive Pay," *Business Week* (April 20, 1998): 64–111.

20. "Oxford CEO's Severance on Hold," *American Medical News,* April 20, 1998, p. 1.

13

The Lure of Single-Payer Health Plans and Why They Will Not Work Here

If every other country uses a single-payer plan or some variant of it and they seem to do all right, why not us? If managed care were not the right answer, would this be? In many ways, managed care and single-payer plans are actually similar. Both ration care for financial reasons, both paternalistically "manage" the care of their subscribers even if in different ways, and both use elaborate monitoring methods that endanger privacy.

A single-payer plan means that all health care is governed and paid by a single entity, a government agency of some kind. We discussed in chapter 10 some of the reasons why single-payer is not a good idea, but the issue is so important that it is worth devoting a whole chapter to it. For this I will draw heavily on my own studies and views and a report written by John C. Goodman and Gerald L. Musgrave for the National Center for Policy Analysis, the nonprofit, nonpartisan research center mentioned previously. I will summarize their report entitled "Twenty Myths About National Health Insurance," adding my own views where appropriate. I would recommend reading the full report.[1]

They studied national health plans in a number of countries, including Canada, the United Kingdom, The Netherlands, Germany, New Zealand, Sweden, Brazil, and Chile. All had or were beginning to implement introduction of access to private care, competition, and other reforms that would dilute the degree of single-payer dependency.

While one of the arguments for national health plans is that they distribute health care fairly to everyone, the reality was that in every country that goal was imperfectly achieved and that "the wealthy, the powerful and the sophisticated find ways of moving to the head of the waiting lines, while the poor, the elderly, racial minorities and rural residents wait longer." They show evidence of the inefficiency of government-run services and how most of the countries rely on private insurance, available to the wealthier people, to reduce the strain on the government programs.

The twenty "myths" they describe are as follows:

1. *Myth: Countries with national plans control costs better and spend less per capita than the United States.* Much of the difference is that we are wealthier and choose to spend more since we can afford to. Canada, which is most often recommended as a model we should follow, is usually thought of as controlling costs better. The actual figures belie this, because Canada's rate of increase has been the same as ours. The often-noted difference in percent of Gross Domestic Product (GDP) spent on health care, Canada's being lower than ours, is a misleading statistic because Canada's GDP has been increasing much faster than ours.* Some of the difference in levels of spending is explained by accounting variations between the two countries. Also, additional expenses for the United States include huge research and development costs Canada does not share (but benefits from as new technology becomes available), higher cost of caring for an older population, many more social problems that entail high expense, such as much higher rates of AIDS, violence, children born to young teenagers, and so on.

2. *Myth: Although we spend more than other countries, our health care is no better.* These claims are based on the fact that crude general mortality rates and infant mortality rates are higher in the United Sates than in many other developed countries. In every country, those rates are lower in the more affluent areas of large cities and much higher in poorer, more rural, or otherwise less advantaged localities. Mortality figures for large populations are dependent almost entirely on social factors, such as AIDS, violence, and teenage pregnancy, that are little influenced by doctors and hospitals. When the United States is compared on measures of actual health care such as care of heart disease and cancer, the United States is at the top. Lifesaving technology is so much more available in this country than any other that there is no

---

*Percent is a fraction, in this case expenditures divided by GDP. If expenditures increase at the same rate, but the denominator, GDP, increases much faster in Canada, their fraction will get smaller, thus making Canada's percentage of GDP look less than it is.

comparison. Some would claim that we overdo technology and procedures and that much if not most is unnecessary. Hogwash! I began in medicine at the start of the modern technological era and saw medicine before and after. Give me after anytime! I give thanks every day for my patients as I make full use of new diagnostic and treatment options and await every new one I can get with great anticipation. Patients now live despite diseases they would have quickly succumbed to without modern technology and quality of life is tremendously improved by modern methods. Failing hearts, livers, and kidneys; previously hidden tumors; cancers that used to be hopeless; strokes that used to be irreversible—the list is endless. Quality of life is equally important and there also we excel. A colleague of mine who is Canadian, but lives and works here, tells me that patients in Canada who are denied needed coronary artery procedures may survive as long, thus making mortality figures seem equal, but they suffer more pain and weakness. Many lifesaving treatments are denied to patients in the United Kingdom based on such factors as age over sixty-five years. Age sixty-five is *young* today. The critical differences modern medicine can make for individuals will not be reflected in crude measures of the entire population of a country.

3. *Myth: There is a "right" to health care in countries with national health insurance.* That right is neither enforceable nor accomplished. Many needed procedures and treatments are delayed so long in those countries that they are in effect denied, or they allow conditions to worsen unnecessarily and patients suffer. This situation in Canada has gotten much worse with severe budget strains exacerbating conditions.[2]

4. *Myth: National plans are more efficient.* Anyone who thinks government programs are more efficient than nongovernmental ones has obviously not observed a Veterans Administration hospital or a municipal hospital clinic as I have. Goodman and Musgrave report show how inefficiency is widespread in countries with national programs. Hospital stays are much longer than ours, they have many more empty beds, and in general their facilities are not run using the modern equipment and techniques that characterize the U.S. system.

5. *Myth: National health plans mean everyone has equal access to health care.* In practice this is far from true. The report shows how in the United Kingdom, Canada, and other countries wealthier people get more, poor and minorities get less, with differences as great as thirty-five times for some services.

6. *Myth: National plans distribute care according to need rather than ability to pay.* It is unlikely that any law can counteract the stronger rule that money talks. Even in situations where a wealthier person cannot exercise influence, privatization and traveling to the United States provide a way for wealthier people to buy more care regardless of restrictions that apply to the less fortunate.

7. *Myth: National plans maintain a high quality of health care.* As noted above, they do not maintain the high level of advanced care that we have in this country. This study and the recent *Business Week* article[3] describe numerous ways that patients with cancer, heart disease, and other problems suffer death or injury due to delays (such as deaths in patients waiting endlessly for bypass surgery), lack of equipment, technology confined to a few special centers, and inefficiencies.

8. *Myth: National plans do fewer "unnecessary" procedures.* The evidence that unnecessary treatments and procedures are common in the United States is based on studies that show differences in treatment of similar patients in different localities and an alleged lack of benefit to the patients who have more done to them. This is an extremely questionable thesis to begin with, since it is based on assumptions and inferences and presumes to be sure that all the patients are comparable. Even if it is correct, other countries, such as Canada and the United Kingdom, have the same disparity by location. If it is true of the United States, it is true for the others as well, and so they are no better at reducing allegedly unnecessary procedures.

9. *Myth: National plans have lower administrative costs.* Some of the difference is in accounting methodology. In Canada, global budgets (lump sums) are assigned to be used at the discretion of local authorities. This may be cheaper but it also reduces oversight of utilization. Even more telling is that most of the excess administrative cost in the United States is due to Medicare, Medicaid, and managed care, which impose huge bureaucratic burdens on doctors.

10. *Myth: National health care is better for the elderly.* That is not the case in the United Kingdom, Germany, France, and Italy, where public policy clearly favors younger people by denying much more care to the elderly than to the young. Kidney dialysis and heart surgery are much less likely to be given to people over sixty-five in other countries compared to here. Proponents of national plans argue that life expectancy is longer in other countries. That is a poor measure, since it is greatly influenced by social factors such as premature deliveries in

young teenage girls (infant deaths reduce longevity figures disproportionately because they occur so early in life) and many others. A better comparison is longevity in later adulthood, for which medical care makes the major difference; by this measure the United States is a world leader.

11. *Myth: Racial minorities fare better under national plans.* There is certainly no guarantee of that and Goodman and Musgrave show how native peoples in Canada and New Zealand fare far worse than the dominant populations.

12. *Myth: Rural areas do better under national plans.* Once again, the assumption is not supported by facts, as there are severe disparities between care available to urban versus rural inhabitants in Canada, the United Kingdom, Brazil, and other countries.

13. *Myth: National plans are better for members of labor unions.* The authors show how the cost of national insurance in the United States would raise the taxes of the middle- and lower-middle-income people to a punishing level. Furthermore, employers would experience such a higher tax burden per worker that jobs in highly unionized industries like automobiles would undoubtedly experience major cutbacks in union jobs.

14. *Myth: National health insurance would make us more competitive internationally by removing the cost of health insurance from the cost of an automobile or other product.* This is a spurious argument for many reasons. First of all, health insurance premiums do not raise salaries. Besides being deductible for the employer, and besides keeping their workforce healthier and therefore more productive, health benefits are just salary given in a different way; if removed, wages would increase to compensate. For example, General Motors is doing better today despite higher health insurance costs because they learned how to make better cars that could compete with the Japanese on quality.

15. *Myth: National plans allocate resources better.* The study shows that they clearly do not. While delaying vital care as noted above, national plans promote popular but less critical things like ambulance transportation for nonemergencies in the United Kingdom (and the ambulances often lack modern equipment). In Canada, there are plenty of primary doctors but a shortage of specialists. National plans are more subject to political pressures—the party in power must please the electorate to be re-elected. Since serious disease affects only a small percentage of the population at any one time, the less critical crowd-pleasers that affect

large numbers of people get more attention, even though they may be of lower medical priority. Those services may be of real value, such as doctor visits for minor colds, home care, and social services, but not at the price of taking less care of serious illness. If people had to pay their own money for minor things like small lacerations and colds, then public money could be better preserved to treat cancer and heart disease in these systems, and, in fact, in any system.

16. *Myth: "Free care" encourages preventive medicine, which lowers costs by keeping people healthier.* In the long run that is probably true, but in the short run preventive medicine is expensive and raises costs. Prevention is more than worth what it costs because its benefits are so great; it is worthwhile as health care but not as a method of short term cost control. I pointed out in chapter 2 that a good doctor uses visits for even minor problems to look for ways to enhance the well being of the patient, including prevention. That works well when the doctor has the time and inclination to do so. In national plans, where visits are very low cost to the patient, the doctors are so overloaded that there is no time to do those desirable things.

17. *Myth: National plans will work if they are just remedied a little.* The factors that mold national health plans seem unlikely to change, so reform is unlikely. One of the main reasons is the politics we noted in myth 15. The most successful politicians please the vast middle class where most of the votes are. The poor and the minorities do not have the political power to win equity for themselves and no one is simply going to give it to them. Furthermore, tough rationing decisions are political suicide. "Elect me because I will save money to provide Band-Aids for your cuts by saving money on kidney dialysis, though unfortunately that will allow nine thousand kidney failure patients to die who could have been treated." That kind of decision, which is representative of what actually happened in the United Kingdom, the politicians prefer to leave to faceless bureaucrats.

18. *Myth: People prefer national health insurance.* Goodman and Musgrave cite studies that confirm what we all know to be the case: Americans will not tolerate long waits, restriction on services, and other necessary results of national plans. They will also not tolerate high taxes to pay for such a plan.

19. *Myth: If it is popular in other countries, it will be popular here.* This is difficult to document, but some common sense will answer it. Most countries have never known private medical care, or at least not for a very long time. Furthermore, the evidence of popularity is mainly

from the media, which reflect the vocal minority who are affluent and benefit the most. Even if national health care is popular elsewhere, that does not mean Americans will like it, and probably will not for the reasons noted above. It is very risky to extrapolate between cultures. Few would dispute that there are major cultural differences among Germans, French, Italians, Japanese, Britons, and even Canadians, compared to Americans.

20. *Myth: Government is essential to national health programs.* Goodman and Musgrave use this section to explain some critical factors in determining health care planning. First of all, they note that large corporations and groups could create their own global health plans within their groups at their own expense without imposing cost on other taxpayers. A large corporation, like Chrysler in their example, could set up a plan similar to the Canadian system that applies to its own workforce.

More importantly, though, Goodman and Musgrave show how politics is the underlying sculptor of all government-run plans and why that is not good. Politicians are like companies—they must respond to the demands of their customers (voters) to sell their product (get elected). Suppose a politician has access to $5,000 to be spent on his fifty constituents, which would be $100 each. Let us say that a particular voter would want $50 for health care, $30 to help educate his children and $20 toward a tax savings on a retirement plan. The politician wants to come as close to this as possible to win that vote. However, the politician cannot allocate $50 to that one voter for a specific purpose. Instead, he has to devise some health benefit that will in general be a $50 value benefit to each of one hundred voters. If the individual voter does not need or want that benefit, it is of no value to him. If the voter could spend the $50 in any way he wished, he would spend it on what *he* needed, not what was allocated in some general plan. Thus when politicians—or managed care executives—spend *your* money in ways *they* think you need, you are often the loser. Your vote does not make that much of a difference because politicians tend to sell the same product since they are appealing to the same large group of voters. If they could design benefits for each individual, the process would work much better, but obviously that is impossible.

Likewise, the desire for votes leads to the better-represented getting more than the needy because the latter have less clout and less ability to deliver votes.

There are other reasons Goodman and Musgrave cite that explain differences between the United States and the United Kingdom, such as studies that have shown that Americans would rail against much of the kind of care given in the United Kingdom but for which the British feel very grateful. We expect much more. Culturally and because of a long history with the National Health Service, people in the United Kingdom do not expect anywhere as much as we do. They also perceive their health system as a "free" service for which they are willing to sacrifice. The huge tax burden makes it anything but free, but that does not seem to affect their perception of it as a free benefit they should be grateful to have.

The United Kingdom seems to endorse the caring versus curing philosophy similar to that of Victor Fuchs, which we discussed in chapter 2, in which doctors are reserved just to cure and less expensive people do the "caring." When asked what they would do with more funds, British health planners said they would put it into "services for the aged, the chronically ill and the mentally handicapped." While those are admirable purposes, they seem lower in priority to saving lives with kidney dialysis machines, heart surgery, modernization of hospitals, and the like.

Government bureaucracies work by delegating power to smaller bureaucratic elements down the line. The problem with bureaucracy is that too often its primary purpose becomes the protection of its own power and perks, usually requiring action and procedures that may be contrary to the needs of those the bureaucracy is supposed to be serving.

One further impact of politics is the same as what happens in corporations. For corporations, profits may be reduced if investment is made for the future, but stock performance is often related to current results, not potential. Likewise, voters may not perceive the value of capital spending to replace aging infrastructure such as hospitals. That may explain why there is such a lag in the United Kingdom and government hospitals in the United States.

NOTES

1. John C. Goodman and Gerald L. Musgrave, "Twenty Myths about National Health Insurance," NCPA Policy Report no. 128, December 1991, http://www.publicpolicy.org/~ncpa/studies/s166/s166.html.

2. Joseph Weber, "Canada's Health-Care System Isn't a Model Anymore," *Business Week,* August 31, 1993, p. 36.

3. Ibid.

14

A Better Way

Everything should be made as simple as possible, but not simpler.
—Albert Einstein

I believe that I have shown that managed care is an unacceptable health care system. It does not accomplish its goals; it destroys the crucial doctor-patient relationship; it creates untenable ethical conflicts for physicians; it allows only minimal, easily counted care at the expense of much needed care for serious illness; and it does nothing to help the uninsured. *Your* health must not be someone else's investment! What is important for you may be bad for that person's investment—your needs must come first.

The Commonwealth Fund recently carried out a major study of physicians' experience with managed care which confirms that doctors are finding all the problems I have been describing.[1] They find time with patients reduced, difficulty in getting needed tests and consultations with specialists, impaired continuity of care, and time to keep their knowledge up to date is more limited. They report severe ethical conflicts inherent in the process, including financial incentives that are contrary to the needs of patients. Their autonomy has been eroded and they are burdened with excessive administrative overhead, financial strains, and excessively long hours. Not only will patients suffer the longer this continues, the demoralization of those physicians whose lives are dedicated to doing good will undoubtedly have serious repercussions.

Why not just improve managed care? I believe I have successfully demonstrated that managed care is inherently unethical. If one corrected its faults, it would no longer be managed care. If we allow others to turn health care into their investment, then the money paid for insurance is allocated to maximize the investors' benefit rather than the patients'. I believe your money should go to your health care, not to someone else's financial return. The argument that others must "manage" health care for us is paternalism of the worst kind and contrary to our concept of self-determination in this country. Making expert advice available if wished for is appropriate; forcing us to have someone else make your decisions is contrary to our principle of freedom. The hope that investors will somehow become altruistic is unrealistic. Investors and the managers the companies employ are far removed from any direct knowledge of the effects of their actions.

Dr. Bernard Lown, Professor of Medicine at Harvard and one of the cofounders of the organization International Physicians for the Prevention of Nuclear War, which won the 1985 Nobel Peace Prize, is also a cofounder of the Ad Hoc Committee to Defend Health Care, a group of health professionals who want a moratorium on further changes in health care until there can be a real debate on how we should proceed.

The Ad Hoc Committee held a meeting on December 2, 1997, after a mock "Tea Party" in which they threw symbols of managed care abuses into Boston Harbor as an echo of the original Boston Tea Party. When he opened the meeting, Dr. Lown expressed that he also felt that managed care could not be reformed and gave as illustration the following parable, which I will phrase in my own words:

> A scorpion said to a toad, "I cannot swim and I must cross the river. Will you give me a ride on your back?"
>
> The toad answered that he was not crazy enough to do that because the scorpion would sting him and he would die.
>
> The scorpion said that there was no logic in that. "If I sting you, you will drown and take me with you, so you know I will not sting you."
>
> The toad thought about it and decided that that made sense and took the scorpion on his back and began to take him across the river. Halfway across, the scorpion stung the toad.
>
> As the toad was dying and they were both slipping below the waves, the toad said, "Where is the logic in that? You have killed us both."
>
> The scorpion answered with its last breaths, "It has nothing

to do with logic. It is my nature to sting and kill and I cannot change my nature."

IF INVESTORS CANNOT RUN MANAGED CARE FOR THE BENEFIT OF PATIENTS, CAN DOCTORS IN PRACTICE ADMINISTER THEIR OWN INSURANCE COMPANY FREE OF OUTSIDE INVESTORS OR EXECUTIVES?

There is a new trend that some predict will take over from managed care companies run by businesspersons: doctors in practice running their own companies. The idea is that the physicians will eliminate the overhead of the outside companies' profit and administration and will be directly responsible for the care of their patients without outside intervention. Common sense should tell us that if a group of business-inexperienced doctors think they can suddenly try to become experts in a highly competitive market, they may be in for a rude awakening. Many who have tried have failed and have had to bring in a managed care company to bail them out.

Even if doctor-run care facilities do better than managed care, they will face the same choices that managed care executives now face. If they set a limit of how much they want to spend in total, they will have to act like a managed care company or fail. If they do not set limits, they will just be a large group of doctors with a corporate name. There may be improvements around the edges and the doctors will find it harder to exert the necessary heartlessness, but the end result is inevitable—fail, or become just like managed care.

In George Orwell's *Animal Farm,* the animals overthrow the oppressive farmers, but in the end, some animals become rulers and the other animals can no longer tell the difference between their animal rulers and their former human ones. Such may be the fate of doctors who think they can escape the inevitable corrupting power of money.

Despite my pessimism, doctors should be encouraged to try running their own insurance companies under today's managed care system. They may do better than the business executives and it may be a kinder, gentler way to manage care.

One of my classmates from medical school, Stephen Hefler, has been working for some years on developing innovative managed care systems in New Jersey that he says are run completely by doctors and patients. He believes they have been successful in establishing procedures that monitor utilization but give doctors and patients much more leeway and a real say in the treatment and reimbursement process.

The Mayo Clinic is said to have built a system where a group practice with fixed, prepaid fees works equitably. If they have truly accomplished this, as may have some other clinics, that is wonderful, but these are unique institutions developed over very long periods of time under special circumstances. They are completely doctor-run, but if they become too big, it is unlikely that they will be able to retain the qualities that allow them to deliver ethical care.

These programs are laudable efforts to achieve the best compromise between two worlds. If there were no better way, they would be our best answer. What concerns me is that the doctors still serve two masters and, if financial pressures mount, the patients will again pay the price.

Another option is to expand Medicare and Medicaid. I think government cannot change its nature either. If you build it, they will come and make it too big. Each bureaucrat, however well-meaning, will add just one more thing, one more control, one more regulation, until we are buried in procedure, detail, and restrictions. Taxes would shoot up dramatically as the cost of care skyrockets. As government programs already in place run out of money, they impose increasingly restrictive changes in an unsuccessful effort to stay within budget.

Both managed care and government programs mean that someone else is telling you how to live your life and what you can and cannot have. They will allow you less and less time with your doctor; you will lose even more of your privacy; and you will have less access to care as the escalating budgets require ever more restrictions.

* * *

Monroe E. Trout, M.D., J.D., former chairman of the board of American Healthcare Systems (AmHS), set up a research unit, then called AmHS Institute, while he was at AmHS, and gave it the assignment to study ways to improve health care delivery at reasonable cost.[2] On November 11, 1992, Trout spoke before the Medical Executives group, presenting the report's findings and adding some insights of his own.* Even then he had foreseen many of the problems we now face. He felt that the massive Clinton health care plan was unnecessary because

*I spoke with him recently and he advised me that while the numbers may have changed since 1992, the principles remain valid.

there was so much waste in the current system that we could reduce costs and improve equity without gutting the system then in place. He said that he did not like managed care, but he liked it even less since it had become only managed cost.

Let me summarize some of the report's findings and the thoughts Trout presented that day. In comparison with other countries, the researchers found similar findings to what we discussed in chapter 13. They surveyed over ninety countries and found that health care in the United States surpassed them all. Trout also dismissed the comparisons based on infant mortality, longevity, and the rest because he also felt those differences are due to societal differences, not medical ones. Unit members looked at Canada's national health care system. It had one advantage in that administrative costs were lower, but when they took *all* costs into account, Canada's costs were as high as ours. For example, we have enough people over age sixty-five to account for one-third of the difference in cost. We have a much higher rate of teen pregnancy, abortions, and so on. He also noted that Americans simply would not tolerate the long waits and limited resources available under the Canadian system.

Administrative costs in the United States comprise 25 percent of health care costs. Reducing that cost to 15 percent would have saved $81.7 billion then—and an astounding $117 billion in 1998. Some of the ways the report suggested to save on these costs would be to combine the duplicative Medicare and Medicaid administrations; to eliminate the veterans hospitals, providing veterans better treatment with all the same benefits in regular hospitals; to simplify billing methods; and the like.

Trout expressed that it makes no sense to provide subsidized care for wealthy people under Medicare.

He noted the high cost of lifestyle. The research unit had calculated that it cost the health care system $1.82 for each *ounce* of alcohol consumed. (Americans consumed *6.7 billion gallons* of alcohol in 1996.[3]) The report said that tobacco health costs were pegged then at $54 billion, or $2.00 per pack smoked. It noted that these costs are 9 to 10 times the excise tax paid on alcohol and tobacco.[4] He recommended designating these taxes for health care use only and then raising the tax to equal the health cost, which would generate revenue to pay for the care of those who made themselves ill and would incidentally discourage use of the substances.

Simple prevention is amazingly cost effective. A rubella immunization would cost a few dollars. Caring for one rubella-damaged baby for a lifetime cost $354,000. A drug-addicted baby cost $63,000 for the first five years compared to the low cost of rehabilitating the mother. A liver transplant for an alcoholic patient cost $250,000, compared to the minuscule cost of an alcohol prevention program. Severe head injury, if someone does not wear a helmet or use a seat belt, cost $310,000; caring for a quadriplegic cost $570,000 over a lifetime, a huge amount compared to the cost of the preventive devices. Four hundred dollars' worth of prenatal care can save as much as $400,000 to treat a mother and child if something goes wrong.[5]

Trout noted that the Chrysler corporation had long complained about the cost of health insurance to their bottom line, but at the same time had been among those most in opposition to helmet laws for motorcyclists and bicyclists, which Trout estimated had saved $100 million in just the first eighteen months by reducing expensive head injuries.

Trout estimated at that time that it would cost $26 billion to give access to health care to all then who were uninsured. The savings he suggested would have paid for the insurance plus much more.

There was great interest in the report in Washington at that time, but it soon dissipated in the morass of debate over the Clinton proposal. Had these suggestions and others in the report been put into action, we would be far better off today.

Taking into account all that I have said up to now, based on extensive experience and research, I will outline the following principles that I believe should be the basis for a better health care system than that which we have now:

1. Every citizen must have access to adequate care. That means universal coverage, portable anywhere.
2. The program must adhere to the highest ethical standards, as I have explained them.
3. Any new health care system should be kept as simple as possible. Some federal rules and regulations will be needed, but they should be the barest minimum.
4. Administration of health care should be local. Medical care is too personal for distant administrators to decide. There should be a basic central structure and standards, but as much as possible should be decided locally. The same principle of simplicity should apply locally as well. Welfare programs, for all their problems, work best when administered by state and local governments.
5. There are three ways to earn income: by the sweat of your own efforts, by profiting from the work of others you employ, and

by return on money invested. For medicine, the only correct way is the first—patients paying the doctor directly. No corporations, stockholders, bottom lines, or distant monitors should exist to interfere with care or invade privacy.

6. The first part of this book has made what I believe is a strong case showing why restrictions on care based primarily on cost rather than a doctor's judgment are wrong and counterproductive. They create ethical conflicts and impair care. Therefore, we must avoid such restrictions.
7. We must devise a system with built-in control of excess care that nevertheless preserves ethical standards. In the past, with traditional health insurance providers, the complaint against physicians was that they had no incentive to limit the services they provided because the more they prescribed, the more they earned. The patients did not want any limits because they paid only a small portion of the bill—the insurer paid the rest.
8. The only way to limit costs and yet retain patients' control of their own lives is to make the patient responsible for choosing the level of care for which they are willing to pay. That means every encounter must involve enough cost to the patient to ensure thoughtful selection, though not so high that it would limit needed care.
9. Physician fees for visits and consultations must not be controlled other than by patient choice based on their own budget decisions as to what they can afford, and competition between doctors to attract patients. Price controls distort markets and are counterproductive. Imposing fee controls inevitably leads to restrictions on patient visits which steal the time that should be available to patients.
10. Patients must be in charge of their own care and their own lives.
11. Physicians and nurses must be free to practice their professions to the fullest level of quality and ethical standards and for the sole benefit of the patient. They must be able to charge fees in an open market subject to the same market forces as anyone else.
12. Patients must have sole discretion as to who has access to their records, other than by court-ordered subpoena or for vital public health protection.
13. The best medical care is given by doctors and nurses as individuals tending to the people of their own communities. Solo practice has the advantage that the physician has complete

control. Small groups can function almost as well, without compromising the autonomy of the member doctors, and they provide some relief in coverage and some efficiencies of size. When groups get too large, however, it is no longer a few doctors working closely together. It becomes a business with all the encumbrances that business brings to professional endeavors. Such expansion needs to be curtailed, perhaps by tax barriers to groups above a certain size.

We must also discourage hospitals and practice management companies from buying doctors' practices. They put the doctor on salary and control every aspect of the practice. A small group of nonprofit centers, such as the Mayo Clinic, the Cleveland Clinic, the Lahey Clinic, and others, are obvious exceptions.*

14. The central governments, state and federal, are very important to set certain basic standards, coordinate major services, and protect basic rights. A strong barrier must be drawn between these functions and the patients' authority over their own lives.
15. Means testing is essential to determine each patient's ability to pay so that *premiums,* not prices of services, are fairly and reasonably set for each person. It should count *all* income, taxable or not, as well as liquid assets (investments, bonds, etc., as opposed to your house or car) above amounts that are reasonable for financial security.
16. The problem of the very high-cost procedures, such as transplants, prolonged ICU stays, extremely premature babies, and the like, must be addressed directly. There will probably have to be some sort of endowment fund, whose source will have to be devised, that will kick in beyond any other coverage. Criteria for using this fund will have to be set by an independent agency with an administrator who is held accountable (see below). There should be local and regional input. Since there will be no profit motive in the decisions and those making the decisions will not have a conflict, it will have greater legitimacy.
17. We must keep administrative functions simple and efficient.

*These are high-quality institutions of great value. They are, in effect, outpatient teaching hospitals and are major contributors to education and research. They are the models that managed care was supposed to follow, but it was totally unrealistic to think that their success could be applied more widely. They grew from long tradition and exist as exceptions that prove the rule.

18. Medicine is getting so complex that we must find new ways of keeping doctors and nurses current and effective. Technology will help by innovative ways of bringing current educational information quickly to doctors, nurses, pharmacists, and patients.
19. Medical care must *not* be governed by guidelines, clinical directives, or committees. Any administrative entities I recommend are each to be headed by a single individual who will decide for him- or herself, but this must be someone who will will stand up and take responsibility for those decisions.
20. Doctors and nurses deserve and should receive the respect and autonomy they have earned, as they in turn should show the highest respect for their patients and should preserve the patients' autonomy just as they want for themselves.
21. New technology is needed to reduce medication errors, drug interactions, and other sources of potential harm.
22. Malpractice is a thorny problem. While most awards are well under $1 million, there are enough above that level to create a threat that has a chilling effect on the way good doctors practice medicine. Malpractice adds to the high cost of medicine directly by the cost of insurance, litigation, and awards, and indirectly by driving doctors to practice defensive medicine. As we have noted, as medicine has become a highly technical field, juries no longer have the expertise to evaluate the conflicting claims of plaintiff and defendant. Juries are also subject to emotional appeals for sympathy for injured people and they may award large sums thinking that it is just insurance company money and the poor plaintiffs deserve help. The current system works poorly for everyone, even for the successful plaintiffs, whose awards are often reduced by judges and are always long delayed by appeals and the slow pace of judicial proceedings. As we noted in chapter 10. ERISA moves claims against HMOs into the federal court system, where juries tend to make more modest awards. If Congress could help the federal system develop ways to provide sensible remedies for plaintiffs that are fair to defendants, that might solve the problem. Some states, like California, are simply limiting malpractice awards, but plaintiffs' attorneys feel that is unfair to them and their clients. An alternative to the federal courts and caps on awards might be to set up an independent arbitration system of some kind. In addition, there should be an agency devoted purely to research and education of all involved to find and reduce causes of malpractice.

23. We must develop new ways of protecting privacy as we increase dependency on computers.
24. We need to develop better service to rural areas, inner cities, the poor, and the homebound. This will require a new commitment to the poor, and ways to reach people in isolated areas, including computer hook-ups and enhanced helicopter services.
25. We must increase support to our great medical centers, since there is no better investment than medical education and research.
26. People should be free to choose any physician.
27. Every citizen must have health insurance of some kind. No one should be able to opt out of paying, putting a greater share of the cost on fellow citizens, only later to come demanding care when they become ill.

How can we meet these goals and requirements? I would propose the following as a framework for discussion. I do not pretend that these are the only or the best answers, but I believe they satisfy the principles I have just outlined. Any alterations to these proposals should still satisfy those principles.

The purpose of these proposals is to design a plan that (1) ensures that *every* citizen has at least adequate care, and the option for better; (2) makes every patient responsible for part of the cost so that patients themselves set limits and normal market forces are brought into the process for the first time; (3) ensures that all citizens choose their care, according to their ability to pay; (4) ends intrusion into patients' private lives and records; (5) simplifies administration; (6) ends micromanagement and wasteful duplication; and (7) frees employers from the burdens.

RECOMMENDATION FOR A NEW HEALTH CARE SYSTEM FOR AMERICA

The United States population is quite diverse. Currently Americans are subject to a wide hodgepodge of coverage. No system can meet the needs of every segment with exact equality. Government-run systems do not. They are designed by politicians needing voter support and are geared toward the healthy members of the middle class, where the bulk of votes is, and toward the affluent class, where most of the campaign contributions and power come from. Managed care is designed primarily for the benefit of large corporations and its purpose is maximizing return on investment. Less favored in this distribution of health care are heavy consumers of health care who cannot afford large out-of-pocket payments, the poor, members of groups subject to discrimination, such as Native Americans, and those who might be isolated geographically or by inner city poverty.

If we are to design a better system that will come closer to serving the entire society, let us first characterize the groups whose needs we must meet.

First are the poorest poor, those for whom spending even a few dollars is difficult, such as single welfare mothers in the inner cities, their children, homeless people, Native Americans whose reservations do not have oil or casinos, and the elderly whose Social Security check is their only income. Members of this group usually qualify for Medicaid, if they know enough to apply for it, and, if over sixty-five, Medicare, if they can afford the premiums and deductibles. They can afford little beyond what these programs pay for.

Next are those with-low paying jobs or at least some savings and the elderly who subsist solely on Social Security, all of whom, along with the poorest poor, comprise the bulk of those on Medicaid rolls (Medicaid eligibility varies by state, is based on factors like income, assets, and number of dependents, and generally is intended for people who fall below the federally established poverty level, though by how much varies by state).

The next group up the ladder are those who do not qualify for Medicaid (they have too much income or too few dependents), are too young for Medicare, and have no health insurance. They are uninsured for one of three reasons: (a) they work for employers who do not provide health benefits (the largest group), and cannot afford health insurance on their own, (b) are unemployed, or (c) choose not to purchase insurance in favor of other uses for those funds. These are the 42 million (as of 1998 estimates) uninsured Americans, of whom more than 10 million are children. Most uninsured people remain so for only a short time, but probably 12 to 15 percent are continuously uninsured for one to two years or more. While uninsured, people receive inferior health care.[6] The cost of providing all of the uninsured with coverage was estimated at $19.9 billion in 1994.[7]

The next group up is the largest, the majority of Americans who work and whose employers provide health insurance as a benefit. Some employers provide health insurance at no cost to the employee, whereas others will pay part of the premium and the employee pays part. Since it is group coverage, the rates are very favorable compared to what self-employed individuals currently pay for the same coverage. The portion of the premium paid by the employer is nontaxable income to the employee, which can be worth as much as 50 percent more in saved federal, state, local, and payroll deduction taxes (such as Social Security and Medicare). Because the employer pays for all or much of the insurance as an employee benefit, the employer chooses the insurance. Most employers today offer only managed care insurance.

Corollary to this group are employed people who make the same income but are *self*-employed. Unless they can figure some way to contrive themselves into a group, the insurance premiums for individuals are currently at least twice what they are for members of a group. (A man who has no employees, other than himself, could hire his wife and child to make a group of three, but that would cost additional payroll taxes, make his child pay income tax, and impose additional bookkeeping burdens.)

Next are those who qualify for specific government programs. Veterans are covered by benefit programs of their own and are eligible for free treatment in federal facilities. Military programs cover active military personnel and other federal insurance programs cover nonmilitary federal employees. States may have programs for their employees.

At the top of the heap is the lucky minority for whom money is no object. Insurance coverage or not, they can purchase whatever care they need.

Superimposed on this structure is Medicare. It applies equally to all segments of the population over sixty-five (and some disabled people) who have paid payroll taxes that cover hospital care and all those eligible who elect to pay the modest premiums (compared to non-Medicare insurance) for coverage of physician and other nonhospital bills. The wealthiest American over sixty-five is entitled to the same Medicare benefits as the poorest, since the payments both made were nonvoluntary payroll deductions. Medicare beneficiaries have considerable out-of-pocket costs, which include premiums, deductibles, copayments, medication costs, and noncovered expenses. Money paid into Medicare in the past has been loaned out by the government and Medicare reimbursements for beneficiary's current bills are paid from current payroll deductions, interest, and general revenues if needed.

Next, let us consider a typical HMO insurance plan. A common premium for a family in New York is $7,000 per year for a standard HMO insurance policy that includes the option to obtain health care outside of the insurer's approved network (called POS coverage, this option has much higher out-of-pocket costs than does the same service obtained from doctors within the HMO's network). Even if the employer pays the entire premium, the family is in effect paying $7,000 for the insurance, because the employee's compensation is the total value of salary plus benefits. In other words, the $7,000 is real money whether it goes to the employee directly or to the insurance company to pay for the insurance. (The one difference is as a benefit it is non-taxable.)

Suppose the family has a very healthy year and they have only seen three doctors in their HMO's network, for which the insurance has paid $500 in medical bills. The family's cost for the year is $7,030, of which $7,000 is premiums and $30 is for copayments (at each visit to a network doctor, the patient has to pay a small amount, such as $10). Putting tax considerations aside for now, that means that they spent $7,030 to pay for $500 in bills. The insurance company keeps the unused $6,500 from their premiums (the $7,000 they paid in minus the $500 the insurance company paid out). Their choice of doctor was limited, their decisions on what care they wanted were subject to someone else's disapproval, and their medical record could have been read by an anonymous insurance company functionary.

Now suppose they had not taken out insurance. They would have had their $7,000 to use as they wished, they would have had full freedom of choice of doctor and treatment, and their privacy would have been protected, at a total cost of, say, $800 (since the doctor fees, not be limited by managed care, might have been higher, but they would have gotten more time with the doctor). Since they would have been spending money directly from their own pocket, they would have consulted a doctor only after careful consideration of their need versus the cost, something that would not have been a concern under the insurance plan.

Thus, the family would have to spend more than $7,030 (the cost of the insurance and the copayments) of their own money before the insurance even began to pay more than it cost them (not counting tax factors). If they had a very bad year with very high medical bills that exceeded the $7,030, then the insurance would have been a good deal. That is the way insurance is supposed to work. It is meant to be there when needed for major calamities. We buy life insurance and pay for it for many years to provide for our families if we die, hoping we will not get to use it for a very long time. We insure our house, but we do not use insurance to cover a meal that was burned or a bicycle that breaks down or many other travails of daily life. Yet, we may run to a doctor for a cold or a minor cut. We should use insurance to protect us from major losses. It makes no sense to pay for expensive insurance to cover minor expenses. Yet that is exactly the opposite of what managed care insurance does. It covers you for every little expense, but becomes increasingly restrictive as you need care that is more expensive.

Furthermore, if you pay (or receive as a benefit) $7,000 per year for insurance for your family, money you cannot get back, you will want every bit of benefit you can get for that money. When your medical bills exceed what you have paid for the insurance, you are not even spending your own money. Is it any wonder that medical costs keep escalating? We all want the best and the most that we can get for money we can't get back or that belongs to someone else. The "someone else" is the insurance company, not your neighbor, even though the insurance company is in effect using your neighbor's money to pay your benefits beyond what you have paid yourself. For example, if we pay $7,000 per year and the insurance company takes off $2,100 for their profit and costs, then any bills you have that exceed $4,900 ($7,000 minus $2,100) must be paid for out of premiums paid by someone else. Note also how much the managed care insurance company is taking out of the system.

We are a lot more careful when we spend our own money directly out of our pocket. We shop around carefully and buy only the best car we can *afford* because we are spending our own money, but imagine what you would choose if your very wealthy uncle told you just to pick out whatever car you wanted.

Suppose that instead of your employer paying for your insurance, you did, with your own money. You would keep the money in a special bank account that would preserve the tax advantage you would have had if the insurance was an employer benefit. In return for the tax advantage, you would be permitted to use the money *only* for medical purposes. With only that one condition, you and you alone would decide how that money was spent. If you did not spend it, it would be *your* money to keep for the next year, not the insurance company's to keep for themselves, and it would remain yours until you spent it for medical bills or willed it to your heirs. If you had a good year and did not use much, you might put less in the following year, thus reducing your expenditure. When you pay for full insurance, you pay the full amount every year even when you are doing well. You would still need insurance for catastrophically high bills that would exceed what you could afford to keep in your account, but such insurance would be far less expensive and could be administered much more simply than current insurance. Your employer would no longer tell you what kind of insurance you could have.

Removing insurance as an employee benefit would make sense only if the employer were obligated to make up in salary what you lose in benefits. For example, if you earn $40,000 per year and get health insurance for which your employer pays $5,000, your new salary would be $45,000 without a health benefit. You would now have to pay taxes on the salary you would now earn directly, in our example the extra $5,000, so you would lose that tax benefit. That tax loss would be mostly compensated by making your contributions to your medical savings account (MSA) and payments for the catastrophic insurance, which would be allowed to be made from *pre*-tax dollars; in other words, it would be deductible from the income used to calculate your tax (whether you itemize or not). In this example, if you put $3,000 of the extra salary into your MSA and used $2,000 to pay the catastrophic insurance premiums, none of that $5,000 income would be taxable. The money in the account would continue to be tax-free, as would any interest that accrued, as long as you withdrew it only for medical expenses. Medical use could be easily documented by using a debit card or special checks for all medical bills. The money could be withdrawn for major emergencies, but at the price of loss of the tax benefit and a penalty, similar to early withdrawal of an Individual Retirement Account (IRA).

The employers would be paying the same salary in total, but they would benefit considerably from reduced bookkeeping and management expenses. The salaries they could offer would be higher in dollar amount, thus making them more directly competitive on salary instead of health benefits. They would also be free of the problems that employee unhappiness with managed care brings them.

The National Center for Policy Analysis, which says that it originated the idea, has been promoting MSAs for a long time. They have studied them in Singapore, where they have been long used, and variations of it in corporations like Quaker Oats, Golden Rule Insurance, and International Paper. Several states including Colorado, Mississippi, and Missouri have experimented with them.[8] Medicare has started a pilot program authorized by the Health Care Portability and Accountability Act of 1996 (the Kennedy-Kassebaum bill) which will permit 750,000 Medicare subscribers to try a limited form of MSA.[9]

Why not just take out high deductible insurance? Would not that be the same as using an MSA? The answer is that it would not for many reasons. First is that you would not have the benefit given you as extra salary if just a few employees chose not to use their health insurance benefits, and employers would not be compelled to make it up if many tried to do so. (In my proposal, the employer would be *obligated* to make an exact exchange of salary for the cost of the premiums.) There would be no preferred tax benefit as is achieved in the MSA. Also, for self-employed people now, such a sort of self-insurance with catastrophic back-up is an option, but, unfortunately, high deductible policies currently are expensive and limited, since they apply to a small, higher risk pool of subscribers.

NCPA delineates answers to many questions about MSAs.[10] Would people spend the money wisely? Their results indicate they would. Would it stimulate doctors and hospitals to be more responsive to patient needs and to make their charges clearer and more reasonable? They indicate that they would. Would it help reduce overutilization of health resources? They feel they can show that they would.

To satisfy yourself, look at the website, but with MSAs so limited in use now, any true analysis awaits widespread use. The Medicare MSAs have many restrictions that may reduce their value. However, in this case, I think a convincing argument can be made by just using common sense. Most medical expenses would fall within the amount saved in an MSA. An MSA gives you complete freedom to choose your own health care, it reduces by far the number of people with access to your records, it encourages you to think carefully about what you do to yourself medically, and it restores a normal doctor-patient relationship. Doctors will return to serving your needs without concern about outside intervention or incentives that act against your interests. The doctors and hospitals must please you or you will go elsewhere, since you are now in charge, not the insurance company. If you do not need as much health care in any year, you retain the money that would have been lost to the insurance company. Any monies you do not use grow faster in your MSA than elsewhere because it is tax-free. In fact, for all but major bills, for middle income and above, this is as close to an ideal solution as we are likely to come.

Of course, it is a bit more complicated than this. What about bills that exceed the value of your MSA? For that, you would have catastrophic insurance. Such insurance has a very high deductible. In other words, it does not begin to cover any bills until an amount equal to the deductible has been spent. You would select a deductible that would equal the amount in your MSA. If your MSA has $3,000 in it, your insurance policy would have a $3,000 deductible. The question then arises, aren't we back where we started? Managed care covers less expensive items easily but examines larger items much more carefully to ensure that they are appropriate. Would not catastrophic insurance examine expensive items just as critically?

I believe we can solve this by structuring the system differently. The catastrophic insurance would be a regulated utility. Unlike the managed care companies, it would be nonprofit and would not have their expensive overhead. That alone saves as much as 30 percent that would have gone to profit and unnecessary administration. An independent board, with no profit incentive and no global budget, would examine medical costs and set reimbursement levels for each service. For example, a chest X-ray might be set at $75. That would be the amount that the board had determined would be reasonable for the bulk of radiologists so that everyone would be able to get an X-ray at this price. Note that the board would not set the price but rather would discover the price point realistically available for each service. The doctor would not be required to charge this price, but most likely would. A patient could choose to go to a radiologist who charged more, but the additional cost would be at the patient's expense. This way, no one would be prevented by cost from getting an X-ray, but patient choice would be retained and doctors would not be constrained by arbitrary price controls.

A vital component would be that there must be a significant copayment that could not be waived under any circumstances nor covered by any secondary insurance. In our $75 X-ray example, you might have to pay $20 (or less if you qualified for a discount based on ability to pay). This way, every medical purchase would involve enough cost for the patient that they would not seek that service unless they felt they truly needed it. By making the patient the wise shopper, we reduce the need to have any third parties deciding if the doctor's judgment was correct in ordering the test, procedure or treatment. It would be between the doctor and the patient to decide what is best for the patient. Rather than a global budget, the rate board would set premiums commensurate with estimates based on the costs of procedures. Adjustments could be made yearly based on the prior year's experience. Since the patient's participation in financial risk is now built into the process, it is far less likely that there would be runaway inflation such as occurred when patients had no financial stake in controlling prices.

Is this perfect? Certainly not, nothing is. The wealthier would have less compunction in getting tests regardless of cost, but their excess expenditures would be a small fraction and mostly at their own expense. The system would have to count on the cumulative buying wisdom of all the people instead of allegedly expert "managers." We would have to be careful to avoid the pitfalls of bureaucracy and regulated utilities. I would urge that any such agency have a clearly identifiable head who would be held responsible for the success of the agency with no opportunity to retreat into a committee or faceless bureaucracy. Even if these problems could not be solved perfectly, we would still be much better off than we are now.

There would also be some inequality in tax benefit because the higher the tax bracket, the greater the tax benefit. I feel that will be balanced by the fact that, as we shall shortly discuss, people with lower incomes will need some subsidization. If the inequity is still felt to be too great, tax benefits could be reduced as income rose above a certain level.

The premiums for the catastrophic insurance should turn out to be quite modest, and certainly much less than currently is charged for managed care insurance. This is because (a) there would be tremendous savings in profit and administration; (b) the insurance pool would be so large that premium costs would be lower due to volume; (c) it does not kick in until the high deductible has been met, so the insurance pool is not nickel-and-dimed to death as happens with managed care insurance. Furthermore, the kind of expenses covered would be much more likely to be sought only if really needed. You might run to your doctor for lots of minor things if it only costs you a few dollars, but you are going to think long and hard before you have an operation. Equally important, because this insurance will cover essentially everyone, the pool will be so large that it will be much more cost efficient. That is, the larger the pool of money, the less effect any one bill has. The larger pool can absorb large costs more easily. A decision will have to be made as to whether everyone pays the same or those with riskier health histories pay more (community rating versus experience rating in insurance terms); probably some compromise between the two will prove best.

There are some very large-ticket items that are a sizeable bite for any insurance pool: transplants, care of extremely premature infants who need prolonged intensive care, some adult intensive care cases, some burn treatments, new drugs that are extremely expensive, some types of rehabilitation. A separate fund will be needed for these. The commissioner who heads the insurance pool would administer this as well, with a panel of advisers, local to each area, that would include physicians, clergy, ethicists, and consumer representatives. There are some things where tough choices must be made. I recently referred a forty-year-old patient, whose heart was nearly destroyed by a rare disease, to a major transplant center. They told me that there are twenty patients needing transplants for every donor heart available. I made the best case I could for my patient, but I was glad I did not have to be on the panel that decided who lived and who died. There are only so many donor hearts, but how much we spend on highly expensive treatments for a small number of people is a societal question. Let us hope, as I discussed in the section on how much should we spend on our health, that we keep our priorities in order. I hope that the some of the money society spends on gambling or paying exorbitantly high salaries could be used instead to provide care for a paralyzed child or a new liver for a young mother or the survival of an infant.

As we said, at some point of rising cost, where you cannot pay the entire amount yourself, those who control the money must be involved in decisions that affect your life. I strongly believe that the mechanisms I have just described are so far superior to the way it is done under managed care and Medicare/Medicaid that the choice is obvious.

The next question is that MSAs are fine for employed people and those who are affluent, but what about everyone else? One of the concerns about introducing MSAs into the current system is that they would attract the healthier, wealthier patients, leaving the other forms of insurance to have the much higher cost of the remaining sicker, poorer patients. I would answer this by saying that *every* citizen* in the country (outside of the military) would be under the same system. Then the question is how do we apply this to all the groups I described at the beginning of this discussion.

I believe the answer is clear and simple. Those who are employed at a salary that can support it or who are affluent enough to afford it otherwise would fund their MSA themselves and pay their premiums for their catastrophic insurance. Everyone else who could not afford part or any of it would get a subsidy proportional to their need. Need would be based on assets, debts, income, fixed expenses, and dependents. A self-employed person who in the current system would have been priced out of the market would find it much more affordable to get an MSA/insurance package. Instead of more than double what group rates are, it would be the same (or a little higher under experience rating if there is an adverse health history). Nevertheless, there will be self-employed and lower salary employed people who cannot

---

*Health care of noncitizens, especially illegal aliens, is a major financial drain in a number of states. How their care is handled is a political question, not a medical one. Until it is resolved in some way, a separate fund, administered tightly, is the only way that makes sense.

afford the full cost of funding their MSA and paying the premiums. This would also include most of the currently uninsured, all of the poorest poor, all on Medicaid, and many of the people now on Medicare or under veterans' benefits.

For all these people a fund would be established that would pay as much of the MSA deposit and catastrophic insurance premium as necessary. That would seem to bring us back to government handouts and people spending other people's money. I believe this could be solved by careful means testing of those requesting discounts. That would tell us what each person could afford. They would make whatever part of the payment they could. All but the poorest would be required to pay something. The cost to them would be set, as accurately as reasonably possible, at a level at which it would be a significant enough expense to force them to think about each purchase, but not so high as to deter them from seeking help when they need it. Where the fund makes the MSA contribution, the fund would retain ownership of the money, but as an incentive to spend it wisely, the person would keep 20 percent per year of whatever was not spent. The only people for whom this might not be workable would be the very poorest, those who could not afford any financial contribution. This could be handled by having this group subject to supervision by health advisors who would have authority to oversee use of their funds. Unlike managed care, these advisors would be there for the *primary* purpose of improving the care of their clients, not financial gain; avoiding unnecessary expenditures would be an important but secondary concern. (Those same advisers could be available for a modest fee on a *voluntary* basis to anyone else who, for whatever reason they might have, wanted assistance from someone other than their own doctor.) Is this an ideal situation? Of course not. Far better would be to improve the lot of the poorest with education, safer neighborhoods, a stake in ownership of their own homes, and jobs. I won't hold my breath for that to happen, so at least we can help our least fortunate neighbors to get better health care than they currently receive under current government programs.

Veterans truly deserve the thanks of a grateful nation. Veterans' hospitals are no longer the best place for them to get medical care. While some of the hospitals are closely affiliated with major teaching centers, most provide a highly duplicative and inefficient level of care. We could improve veterans' health care and save many billions of dollars if we fold veterans' medical care into the same system as everyone else (turning the teaching hospital-affiliated VA hospitals over to the medical center as a support for research and education). Those saved funds should be used to improve the veterans' lot first and any left over could be used to finance the medical funds.

Medicare and Medicaid would no longer be needed. The savings on administration and waste alone would be enormous. Both of these types of insurance encourage beneficiaries to spend other people's money unwisely and on minor needs while at the same time doing a poor job of helping those with major problems. By changing to the new system, people would be able to allocate their own resources more wisely and specifically to their own needs.

Payroll deductions would be ended for Medicare. The payroll-deducted monies already paid in for Medicare up to the time it is discontinued would be paid out to the MSA of each person, proportional to their lifetime contribution, on a yearly basis in amounts that would spread the payments affordably over time.

Some people would want to refuse to participate, choosing instead to throw themselves on the mercy of others if their gamble on good health loses. That would no longer be acceptable. Anyone who chose not to participate would be taxed a health tax that would fund the pool for the poor. Those who paid that tax would look to that pool for their care. The reason for the tax is that perhaps we cannot force people to participate in insurance, but the government can enforce a tax needed to provide their care. The tax should be equivalent to what they would have paid in the insurance system.

This new system would be so much simpler to administer that we could almost certainly reduce administrative costs from 25 percent of total health expenditures to only 15 percent. If that happened, we would save *$117 billion,* which could fund most if not all of the costs for those who need subsidization. By making people responsible for spending their own money, there would be an immediate brake on excess spending. I can attest to that based on my own experience with many uninsured people. Every item becomes a matter for discussion and careful consideration. "If you can afford this test, it will tell you . . ." "This brand antibiotic is a little better, but if you use this cheaper generic it will be good enough for this particular infection, but you have to be sure you take it four times a day. You must keep to that schedule or it will not work." " I know that this procedure is very expensive for you, but it is the only way we might pick up the cancer early enough . . ."

Major adjustments will be needed. If we extend decent care to everyone, we will need more doctors and nurses. Doctors will have to adjust once again to a new reality, but this time they will be working with and reaching accommodation with their newly empowered patients face-to-face, rather than struggling helplessly with profit-driven distant corporations. Patients will have to adjust to the new responsibility they have for their own health. Doctors will have to carefully educate patients as to the value of visits, tests, and treatments that the patient will now be examining critically.

Patients will have to decide for themselves whether a visit for a simple cold is necessary. On the one hand, most colds just get better, but on the other, there is that long list of other things we listed in chapter 11 that look like a cold. Patients may not realize that risk and either stay home or perhaps see a nurse practitioner, who, as we discussed may not have the skill and training to pick up subtle signs of serious disease. Patients will have to learn that visits for preventive medicine are worth the cost to them.

Every hospital should become nonprofit, as essentially most once were, and government-run hospitals should be converted to nonprofits as well. Some way would have to be found to compensate investors in the for-profit chains for the loss of their investment (perhaps special tax breaks would encourage some to give up their right to their equity). Once converted, all hospitals should be affiliated with a medical center that would have responsibility for setting standards and ensuring good care.

Part of the money invested in health care will have to go to teaching centers to support education and research. Fortunately, uncompensated care would no longer be a burden on the hospitals. The for-profit hospitals established some useful innovations, the best of which can be retained as long as they do not interfere with quality of care.

We will need to integrate technology into medicine to improve communication and education, but first and foremost must be major new laws and technological breakthroughs to guarantee privacy to the best of our ability. Personally, if I could transport us back to precomputer days I would do so because, as much as I love computers, I think our society suffers more from them than we gain; but such a reversal is impossible, so we must make the most of it. I would strongly urge that the Congress approve and the president appoint a cabinet-level commissioner of privacy who will have the assignment and the authority to recommend laws and enforce regulations that will go as far as we can to restore our freedom to be "let alone," in Justice Brandeis's words as quoted in the section on confidentiality.

Assuming that we cannot resist the encroachment of computers on our lives and that we can at least find a way to minimize their potential for abuse, then they can be of great benefit. The cost should not be unusually high as almost all physicians have computerized somewhat and the Internet obviates the need for an expensive network installation. The most important use would be an educational system that would bring to every doctor a stream of medical news and information, immediate access to library and other information and reference sources, advisories from the FDA and other agencies, textbooks, registries of pharmaceutical information, and potential interactions among drugs and more. One of the ways to avoid disparity in quality of treatment by locality would be to have medical schools present their approach to various problems. For example, a program transmitted nationally could show how heart attacks are treated at Johns Hopkins, Stanford, New York University, Columbia, and other top centers. Doctors could then synthesize from these presentations an approach that would work best in their area. In caring for patients, computers would facilitate consultations. Computers now have the capability of transmitting information as it is occurring. X-rays and other test information can be transmitted digitally to distant experts for opinions. It is now possible to actually operate on a distant patient through robotic arms, technology developed for the space station of the future but just as applicable to reach people in remote locations far from a doctor or hospital capable of the surgery needed. Helicopter services are of course an option as well and need to be used far more for remote areas.

There is too much information available to patients. Not only can it be overwhelming and confusing without medical training to understand it in context, much of it is wrong and misleading. Mainstream medicine must find ways to "sell" the message of good medicine to patients bombarded with a cacophony of competing claims.

Of course, the best guide for patients is to have their own doctor. Under the new system, patients can elect to see good doctors who will spend time with them, serve only their interest, and advise them in terms they can understand based on knowing them as whole people.

In this new medical world, we would all get care as nearly equally as one could reasonably achieve. No longer would we be oppressed in a complicated, bureaucratic system of many different competing interests. By eliminating managed care, Medicare, Medicaid, for-profit hospitals, and all the rest, we would be restoring some sanity and simplicity to that which is vital to all of us, our health and its preservation.

NOTES

1. Karen Scott Collins, Cathy Schoen, and David R. Sandman, "The Commonwealth Fund Survey of Physician Experiences with Managed Care," March 1997, The Commonwealth Fund, http://cmwf.org/health care/physrvy.html 8/21/98.

2. AmHs Institute, *Patients First* (Washington, D.C.: AmHs Institute, 1991).

3. John Wright, ed., *The New York Times 1998 Almanac* (New York: Penguin Reference Books, 1997), pp. 290, 332.

4. AmHs Institute, *Patients First.*

5. Ibid.

6. Steven A. Schroeder, "The Medically Uninsured—Will They Always Be with Us?" *New England Journal of Medicine* 334 (April 25, 1996): 1130–33; Paul W. Newacheck et al., "Health Insurance and Access to Primary Care for Children," *New England Journal of Medicine* 338 (February 19, 1998): 513–19

7. S. H. Long, M. S. Marquis, "The Uninsured 'Access Gap' and the Cost of Universal Coverage," *Health Affairs* 13, no. 2 (1994): 211–20.

8. John C. Goodman and Gerald L. Musgrave, "Personal Medical Savings Accounts," National Center for Policy Analysis, http://www.public-policy.org/~ncpa/bg/bg128.html, July 22, 1993.

9. NCPA, "Medical Savings Account Legislation: The Good, the Bad and the Ugly," http://www.public-policy.org/-ncpa/ba/ba211.html, August 19, 1996.

10. Goodman, "Personal MSAs"; NCPA, "MSA Legislation"; and others at the NCPA website, http://www.public-policy.org.

Epilogue

The shining promise of managed care with which we began this book turns out to have been a false hope. I believe there is a better way. I hope that this book will generate much heat and debate. I believe that I have presented a compelling case, but I am sure that nearly every sentence will be disputed.

I believe we should institute all the changes I have suggested, but there are daunting political hurdles. If I succeed only in igniting a reexamination of where we are and where we are headed, I will have at least made a start.

We have drifted into a system in which each of as individuals is gradually losing control of a vital part of our lives—the care of our health. If we wait much longer to act, it will be too late. Our freedoms were hard-won, but they are ever in danger and need constant vigilance to defend. When times seem good, we are lost in our daily routine and the importance of little things. That is the time of greatest peril, because danger often tiptoes in on cat feet.

While we were not looking the normal, banal process of government and business waged a war and won a revolution. No one noticed. There were no sounds of shots or bombs, but the change was as great as if there had been. Why does it matter so much? Besides the fact that it is simply wrong and unfair, you or your family may suffer actual harm. You will have to decide whether you want just to glide along with the flow, hoping you will only have minor problems that need little, or whether you want the security that a real health care system will be there for you when you need it. I believe I have pointed the way to assure the latter.

We do *not* have to surrender our rights to others. We *can* do better.

Appendix

How to Make the Most of an HMO, If You Must Be in One

Managed care is so pervasive that few people have alternatives.

Most Americans under sixty-five today get their health insurance through their employers. Over 85 percent of employers now offer only managed care plans.

Those who want traditional insurance will find that the patient base for these plans has shrunk so low that their premiums are now double what they were before managed care. Individuals who do not get health insurance from their employers and are not part of a group of at least two or more will pay sky-high premiums.

Medical savings accounts are so far available only on a limited basis for Medicare patients. As you may recall, these allow the insured to place their own money in a tax-favored account, which can be used for medical expenses (and a few other purposes) free of any outside controls. Any money not used belongs to the insured, not the insurance company. Under current rules, the insured is obligated to purchase an insurance policy whose deductible is equal to the MSA fund; it kicks in when the MSA money is exhausted. Unfortunately, the secondary insurance is often rather limited and can entail high out-of-pocket costs. Although there is controversy about the impact of MSAs as health care policy, these plans as presently designed are beneficial for high-income individuals.

An alternative is to self-insure your own MSA. Although it would not have any tax benefits, you could put some money into an account that you would use only for medical bills and supplement it with an indemnity insurance policy that would have a deductible equal to your designated account. This would at least have the advantage of total freedom and you would retain the money you did not spend. But you would have to convince yourself to spend those funds when you needed them. We are all so used to having our bills paid partly by health insurance, our sense of expense is distorted. If you spend $2,000 of your own money instead of $5,000 on insurance premiums, you will be much better off, but it will seem expensive to you to be laying out hundreds of dollars for things you used to pay for with insurance and a copayment.

We discussed in the text the reasons our current system has developed as it is and what are its problems. I have proposed what I believe are far better ways than our current system, but politically such changes might be difficult to pass. We may be stuck with the current dismal system for a long time.

How do you make the best of a bad situation?

- If you can afford traditional indemnity insurance, an MSA, or self-funding, do so immediately and enjoy the luxury and freedom it will provide you.
- If your only choice is managed care, then be prepared to fight for what you require and deserve.
- When all you need is brief preventive care or help with minor problems, you will probably find little difficulty. The small copayment and the absence of forms are even easier than traditional medicine, but, of course, you will get the bare minimum of care.
- Furthermore, you should avail yourself of every free option the insurance offers—immunizations, mammograms, and the like.
- The drug plans are helpful as they can significantly reduce your cost for routine medications, though you may not have as full a choice as you would like.
- If you have the option, pick a plan (called a POS) that allows you to see doctors who are not in the HMO network. If available, pick a plan that allows you to go directly to a specialist and that has the fewest restrictions. You must read the contracts in detail and ask questions about the many vague areas.
- Find out how the plans work: whether they are capitation, if there is a withhold or a gag clause, what happens when you are away from home, and so on.
- Make sure you know all the rules, such as preapproval for an emergency room visit, how to get lab work and procedures, etc.
- When you see the doctor, recognize that the doctor is under

great pressure to make the visit as short as possible. Come equipped with a written list of questions and what you want from the doctor. Confine the list to what is most important. The doctor will have little time to spend with you, so the better prepared you are, the more likely it is you will achieve your goals for that visit. Most advice books say that you should be insistent on covering everything on your list, but that you should do so politely because you want to avoid being seen as a "problem" patient.

- Educate yourself on your medical problem ahead of time as much as you can. There are many good books. Stay with the ones from the major medical centers—Columbia College of Physicians and Surgeons, Mount Sinai, Mayo Clinic, the AMA guides, and similar resources. The *Tufts Diet and Heath Newsletter* is excellent and there are good newsletters from Johns Hopkins, *The Berkeley Wellness Newsletter,* and others.

  Books and similar sites on the Internet can be very helpful, but be very careful because there is also much bogus or unsubstantiated information. For example, the fact that there is a website dedicated to a disease does not mean that its information is necessarily valid. Two such diseases that engender a great deal of erroneous and unfounded information are Lyme disease and chronic fatigue syndrome.
- Learn ahead of time the appeal procedures the HMO uses, in case you are denied care you feel you are entitled to.
- Medicare and Medicaid work differently from managed care, but similar principles apply to making them work for you.
- The following books go into considerable detail and are very helpful:
  - Alan J. Sternberg, *The Insider's Guide to HMOs, How to Navigate the Managed Care System and get the Health Care You Deserve* (New York: Plume Books [Penguin Books], 1997)
  - *The Castle Connolly Guide to the ABCs of HMOs, How to Get the Best from Managed Care* (New York: Castle Connolly Medical Books, 1997)
  - Nancy Levitin, *Health Care Rights* (New York: Avon Books, 1996)

Note: I cannot vouch for everything in these books, since as a nonparticipant in managed care, I do not have direct experience in making it work for patients, but they seem to offer sound advice. Managed care and government programs are the reality for most

Americans. It greatly saddens me that we live under a system where patients have to "survive" the health care system, where they have to manipulate, cajole, and demand to receive what should be theirs by right. There is something very wrong when a person has to fear being labeled a "problem" patient simply because he or she requests good care.

I wish you the best success in maintaining health and fitness.

Glossary

This includes some of the terms used in this book, as well as some additional terms of interest. These are brief definitions for the layperson are based on my own knowledge and on the references listed in the bibliography at the end of this book. More detailed or technical definitions can be found in the references.

AARP. The American Association of Retired People, the largest, most powerful lobby for senior citizens.

Allowed amount. The maximum amount an insurance policy will pay for a given service, regardless of the charge for that service.

Ancillary services. Most services not provided directly by doctors, such as laboratory work, physical therapy, and diagnostic studies.

Assignment. If a doctor "takes assignment," it means that the doctor will accept the insurance company's allowed amount as payment in full (the patient may be required to pay part of the allowed amount, called a copayment).

Attestation statement. A written document that physicians must sign to retain hospital privileges. The physician states that providing a false statement in a patient's chart is a federal crime. That physicians are singled out to sign this is insulting and is one of many ways Medicare intimidates doctors.

Balance billing. Billing the patient for more than the insurance company or Medicare allows. Physicians who list themselves as nonparticipating (see below) in Medicare can charge patients a very small amount above the fees set by Medicare. The AARP and other senior groups unfairly characterize this small, completely legal extra charge as "overcharging seniors."

Board Certification. A doctor is said to be board certified if he or she has passed the requirements and exams for a specialty certifying board. The doctor is then a diplomate of the certifying board. A doctor who has met all the requirements but not taken (or passed) the exam is called "board eligible."

Capitation. An insurance plan in which the doctor is paid a set amount per month or year for each patient, regardless of what services are provided to that patient. It is the exact opposite of fee-for-service. In effect, the financial risk is transferred from the insurer to the doctor. The doctor hopes to make more from the patients who require less care than it costs to take care of the patients who need more. If the cost of care exceeds the payments, the doctor loses, not the insurance company. There are three levels of capitation: (a) primary care only, (b) all medical care except hospitalization, and (c) all medical care including hospitalization (known as global risk).

Community rating. An insurance plan in which the premiums are the same for every member of the insured group, regardless of the risk of any of the individuals. Healthy young people pay the same rate as very ill elderly patients. It is the opposite of *experience rating.*

Copayment. The small, set amount that a patient in a managed care contract pays for each visit, procedure, or prescription.

Cost-shifting. This occurs when the costs incurred by one group are charged to another. In the past, hospitals would charge private patients more to cover the cost of care for the poor. Today, managed care has shifted significant cost from the employer to the employee by increasing the total out-of-pocket costs employees pay.

Deductible. The amount per year the insured must pay before the insurance coverage begins.

Diagnosis Related Groups (DRGs). Medicare and some other insurers classify hospital patients into 468 categories. The amount of money allowed for the care of each patient is based on the DRGs (multiple diagnoses are taken into account), not on the specific care provided to the patient. The hospital wins or loses depending on whether they spend more or less than the DRG allowance.

Direct service insurance. The insurer hires doctors and other medical care workers to provide care for their insured. The doctors and others are paid by salary or by predetermined payments. Those who are insured pay a premium which allows them access to the doctors and other services. There is seldom any deductible and there is usually a small **copayment.**

ERISA (Employee Retirement Income Security Act of 1974). This law governs many aspects of private pension and welfare group plans. It is important for managed care because it significantly shields them from much state regulation and from malpractice liability.

Experience Rating. An insurance plan in which each person or group is charged a rate proportional to the risk to incur costs. Age, gender, smoking status, health history, current health, and prior utilization are some of the factors commonly considered in experience rating.

Fee-for-service. The patient pays the doctor a fee for each service rendered. In traditional private practice, the doctor sets the fees. In Medicare and in other insurance plans, the insurer sets the fee.

Formulary. The list of drugs a hospital approves and stocks. In managed care, it is the list of medicines for which the company agrees to pay.

Gatekeeper. As defined by managed care, the patient's primary doctor, who is responsible for planning and coordinating the most effective care for the patient. In practice, it is a way for managed care to reduce costs and limit utilization of more expensive services.

Health Care Finance Administration (HCFA). The government organization that administers Medicare and Medicaid. HCFA 1500 is the standard claim form for physician bills.

Health Maintenance Organizations (HMO). Prepaid health insurance plans in which the patient must use only the services stipulated. HMOs are a type of **direct service insurance.**

Indemnity insurance. Indemnity insurance plans reimburse patients for medical costs according to their own deductible and allowed amounts. The doctor has no relationship to the insurance company and the doctor's only obligation is to the patient.

Independent Practice Association (IPA). Groups of independent doctors, usually organized by HMOs or hospitals, who see patients on a negotiated **fee-for-service** basis. The IPA is paid by an **HMO** on a **capitated** basis.

Informed consent. The obligation to fully inform patients of the risks and benefits of treatment, the nature of the treatment, and reasonable alternatives. As discussed in the text, this is a legal term for what is simply an inherent part of good medical practice.

Long-term care. All maintenance care beyond the acute illness, whether in the hospital, a rehabilitation facility, a nursing home, or at home with assistance. While less expensive on a daily basis, the long duration can pose an enormous financial burden.

Malpractice. *Negligent* medical care, too often confused with an unfortunate outcome due to natural circumstances, simple human error, or the known risk of treatment.

Medicaid. A federal program of health insurance for low-income patients, administered by the states under federal rules and supervision. Administration, structure, and benefits vary from state to state.

Medical Loss Ratio (MLR). The percent of the amount of money, collected as premiums, that is spent on providing the care promised in the insurance contract. The lower the ratio, the less is spent on patient care. HMO profits come from the money not spent on medical care. In the past, before managed care, the MLR has been above 95 percent most of the time. Under managed care, it can be as low as 65 percent.

Medical savings accounts (MSA). A new type of insurance that is in an experimental stage. The basic idea is that tax-deferred money is put in a dedicated savings account to be used for medical costs. A high-deductible insurance policy takes over when costs exceed the funds of the MSA. If the patient puts in his or her own money, then that person retains any money that is not used.

Medical Staff Organization (MSO). A group of doctors who organize to negotiate and contract with managed care plans, most of whom are affiliated with a hospital.

Medicare. A federal insurance plan for people over age sixty-five and those with certain disabilities. Part A is funded by payroll deductions and covers hospital costs. Part B is funded by premiums and covers all other care.

Medigap insurance. Private insurance that pays some of the **out-of-pocket costs** that are not covered by **Medicare.**

Out-of-pocket costs. The amount the patient pays beyond the amount paid by insurance. It includes the **deductible, copayments,** charges in excess of **allowed amounts,** and costs of uncovered expenses. Most plans have a maximum out-of-pocket cost, after which the insurance pays a greater portion of the bill, as long as it includes only allowed procedures.

Participating, nonparticipating. A physician can choose to participate in **Medicare** or not (the choice is made once per year). A participating physician accepts the Medicare-**allowed amount** as payment in full (the patient must pay 20 percent of the allowed amount and Medicare pays the rest directly to the doctor). If a doctor chooses to be nonparticipating, then the doctor can charge above the allowed amount and collect the full fee from the patient. Medicare then reimburses the patient 80 percent of the *allowed* amount. Medicare and the states strictly limit the amount nonparticipating doctors can charge above the allowed amounts. At this point, the states and Medicare have so severely limited fees that there is essentially no difference between participating and nonparticipating. At any point, a nonparticipating doctor can choose to "accept assignment," which means the doctor accepts the allowed amount and is paid the 80 percent directly by Medicare (the patient pays the 20 percent as usual). The **deductible** must always be met first.

Physician-Hospital Organizations (PHO). Joint ventures that provide medical services through managed care plans.

Point of service (POS). Managed care plans that allow patients to see doctors who are not part of the managed care network. When patients go "out of network," they pay a high cost in **deductible,** limited **allowed amounts,** and high **copayments,** as opposed to the much lower cost of seeing in-network doctors.

Precertification. The process of getting approval from the HMO before the hospital admission or procedure is done.

Preferred Provider Organizations (PPO). Groups of independent doctors who have agreed to a discounted, pre-set fee schedule. Patients can choose which doctor they wish to see.

Professional Standards Review Organization (PSRO). Run by doctors, this is an organization that reviews services for **Medicare** and **Medicaid.**

Provider. A term that managed care applies to physicians. I believe it denigrates doctors and distorts patients' perceptions of the physician. The term allows medical care to be treated as just another commodity, which facilitates all the abuses outlined in this book.

Provider-Sponsored Organizations (PSO). Health care organizations owned and run by doctors and hospitals that contract to provide services directly, bypassing managed care companies. They thus save on the cost of the managed care company but assume all of the financial risk.

Resource-based relative value system. An attempt by **Medicare** to give more equal weight to cognitive care and to take into account such factors as doctors' skill, time spent, office costs, and geographic differences. In practice, it significantly reduced fees for surgery and procedures but improved reimbursement for cognitive care and primary care by only very small amounts.

Staff model HMO. An HMO in which care is provided by doctors on salary who work in the HMO facility.

Underwriting. Determining the insurance risk of groups and individuals based on age, gender, health history, smoking, and other factors.

Withhold. Part of the money owed physicians in managed care that is withheld until the year's results are in. If costs meet estimates, the money is paid to the doctors, but if costs are excessive, the money is not paid.

Worker's Compensation Insurance. State-mandated insurance that employers must carry to cover the cost of injury or illness their employees may suffer on the job.

Bibliography

BOOKS AND JOURNALS

Ad Hoc Committee to Defend Health Care. "For Our Patients, Not for Profits, A Call to Action." *Journal of the American Medical Association* 278 (Dcember 3, 1997): 1733–74.

Allen, Arthur. "Medical Privacy? Forget It!" *Medical Economics* 75 (May 11, 1998): 151–66.

Alsop, Ronald J., ed. *The Wall Street Journal Almanac 1998*. New York: Dow Jones Co., 1997.

American Association for Retired Persons. "Out-of-Pocket Costs Are High, Study Shows." *AARP Bulletin* 39 (April 1998): 7.

American Bar Association. *Legal Guide for Americans over Fifty*. New York: Random House, 1997.

American College of Physicians. "Despite Managed Care, Internists Are Satisfied." *ACP Observer* 18 (March 1998): 1.

American Medical Association. *Code of Medical Ethics, 1996–1997 Edition.* Chicago: AMA, 1997.

AmHS Institute. *Patients First.* Washington, D.C.: AmHS Institute, 1991.

Anders, George. *Health against Wealth, HMOs and the Breakdown of Medical Trust.* New York: Houghton Mifflin, 1996.

Annas, George J. *The Rights of Patients: The Basic ACLU Guide to Patient Rights.* Chicago: Southern Illinois University Press, 1989.

———. *Standard of Care: The Law of American Bioethics.* New York: Oxford University Press, 1998.

———. "When Should Preventive Treatment Be Paid for by Health Insurance?" *New England Journal of Medicine* 331 (October 3, 1994): 1027–34.

Asch, David A., and Peter A. Ubel. "Sounding Board: Rationing by Any Other Name." *New England Journal of Medicine* 336 (June 5, 1997): 1668–71.

Blumenthal, David. "Total Quality and Physicians' Clinical Decisions." *Journal of the American Medical Association* 269 (June 2, 1993): 2775–78.

Bodenheimer, Thomas. "The Oregon Health Plan—Lessons for the Nation." *New England Journal of Medicine* 337 (August 28, 1997, and September 4, 1997): 651–55, 720–23.

Bodenheimer, Thomas, and Kevin Grumbach. "Paying for Health Care." *Journal of the American Medical Association* 272 (August 24 and 31, 1994): 634–39.

Bodenheimer, Thomas, and Kip Sukkivan. "How Large Employers Are Shaping the Health Care Marketplace." *New England Journal of Medicine* 338 (April 2 and 9, 1998): 1003–1007, 1084–87.

Brink, Susan. "HMOs Were the Right Rx." *U.S. News & World Report* (March 9, 1998): 47–50.

Burke, Cathy. "Dying Woman Denied Doc She Needs." In "What You Don't Know about HMO's Could Kill You." *New York Post*, September 21, 1995, 15.

Califano, Joseph. *America's Health Care Revolution*. New York: Simon & Schuster, 1986.

Callahan, Daniel. *What Kind of Life: The Limits of Medical Progress*. New York: Simon & Schuster, 1990.

Caplan, Arthur. *Due Consideration*. New York: John Wiley & Sons, 1998.

Carr, A. Z. "Can an Executive Afford a Conscience?" In *Ethics in Practice*, edited by K. R. Andrew. Boston: Harvard Business School Press, 1989.

Compton, Michael T. "My Vocation." *American Journal of Medicine* 104 (March 1998): 317–18.

Cram, David L. *The Healing Touch: Keeping the Doctor-Patient Relationship Alive under Managed Care*. Omaha, Nebr.: Addicus Books, 1997.

Crane, Mark "Medical Convictions." *Reason* (May 30, 1998): 44–48.

Dicker, Fredrick U., and Greg Birnbaum. "Hellish Abuse at City Nursing Homes." *New York Post*, March 15, 1998, 8–9.

Epstein, R. A., D. Lindsay, J. Lally, and U. Reinhardt. "Letters." *Journal of the American Medical Association* 279 (March 11, 1998): 745–46.

Ernst, Edzard. "Harmless Herbs? A Review of the Recent Literature." *American Journal of Medicine* 104 (February 1998): 170–78.

Fein, William S. "The Federal False Claims Act." *Unique Opportunities* (May/June 1995): 9–12.

Finkelstein, Katherine Eban. "The Sick Business." *New Republic* (December 29, 1997): 23–27.

Freudenheim, Milt. "Penny-Pinching H.M.O.'s Showed Their Generosity in Executive Paychecks" *Wall Street Journal*, April 11, 1995, D4.

Fries, James F., et al. "Reducing Health Care Costs by Reducing the Need and Demand for Medical Services." *New England Journal of Medicine* 329 (July 29, 1993): 321–25.

Gibbons, Robert B. "When Housestaff Die: Musings of a Program Director." *American Journal of Medicine* 104 (March 1998): 319–20.

Goodman, John C., and Gerald L. Musgrave. "Twenty Myths about National Health Insurance." NCPA Policy Report No. 128, December 1991, http://www.public-policy.org/~ncpa/studies/s166/s166.html.

"Health Policies Don't Cover Many Expenses." *Wall Street Journal*, January 23, 1998, B7B.

Hergott, Lawrence J. "The Time of Three Dynasties: Reflections on Imbalance in the Practice of Medicine." *Annals of Internal Medicine* 128 (January 15, 1998): 149–51.

Herzlinger, Regina. *Market Driven Health Care.* New York: Addison-Wesley Publishing, 1997.

HIAA. *Managed Care: Integrating the Delivery and Financing of Health Care.* Washington, D.C.: The Health Insurance Association of America, 1996.

Howe, Edmund G., ed. "Managed Care: Patients, Principles, and Politics." *Journal of Clinical Ethics* 6 (Winter 1995).

Hymowitz, Carol. "Psychotherapy Patients Pay a Price for Privacy." *Wall Street Journal*, January 22, 1998, B1, B13.

Isaacs, Stephen L., and James R. Knickman, ed. *To Improve Health Care 1997: The Robert Wood Johnson Anthology.* San Francisco: Jossey-Bass Publishers, 1997.

Jeffrey, Nancy Ann. "Health-Care Costs Rise for Workers at Small Firms." *Wall Street Journal*, September 8, 1997, B2.

Kessler, Jeanne. *Bitter Medicine, Greed and Chaos in American Health Care.* New York: Carol Publishing Group, 1994.

Kilborn, Peter T. "Doctors' Pay Regains Ground Despite the Effects of H.M.O.'s." *New York Times*, April 22, 1998, A1, A20.

Lieberman, Jethro K. *The Litigious Society.* New York: Basic Books, 1981.

Longino, Charles "Beyond the Body: An Emerging Medical Paradigm." *American Demographics* (December, 1997): 14–19.

Macklin, Ruth. *Enemies of Patients.* New York: Oxford University Press, 1993.

———. *Mortal Choices.* Boston: Houghton Mifflin Co., 1987.

"Managed Care 1998." *Medical Economics.* (March 23, 1998): 155–56.

Mechanic, David, ed. *Readings in Medical Sociology.* New York: The Free Press, 1980.

Menikoff, Jerry A. "The Role of the Physician in Cost Control." *Ophthalmology Clinics of North America* 10, no. 2 (June 1997): 191–95.

Menzel, Paul T. *Strong Medicine: The Ethical Rationing of Health Care.* New York: Oxford University Press, 1990.

Millenson, Michael L. *Demanding Medical Excellence.* Chicago: University of Chicago Press, 1997.

Miller, Arthur. *Death of a Salesman.* New York: Viking Press, 1949.

Orient, Jane M. *Your Doctor Is Not In, Healthy Skepticism about National Health-Care.* New York: Crown, 1994.

Packer, Samuel. "Marketing Ethics in Ophthalmology." *Ophthalmology Clinics of North America* 10, no. 2 (June 1997): 211–17.

Packer, Samuel, and George L. Spaeth, eds. "Ethics, Law, and Managed Care." *Ophthalmology Clinics of North America* 10, no. 2 (June 1997).

Pear, Robert. "Clinton Would Broaden Access of the Police to Medical Records." *New York Times*, September 10, 1997, A1, A15.

———. "Health Spending Grew Slowly in '96 but Still Hit $1 Trillion." *New York Times*, January 13, 1998, A15.

———. "New Health Plans Due for Elderly." *New York Times*, June 10, 1998, A1, A26.

Peeno, Linda. "What Is the Value of a Voice?" *U.S. News & World Report* (March 9, 1998): 40–46.

Pelligrino, Edmund D., and David C. Thomasma. *For the Patient's Good.* New York: Oxford University Press, 1988.

Porter, Roy. *The Greatest Benefit to Mankind: A Medical History of Humanity.* New York: W. W. Norton, 1998.

Porter, William G. "Venus on the Right." *Annals of Internal Medicine* 128 (March 15, 1998): 500–501.

Reingold, Jennifer. "Executive Pay." *Business Week* (April 20, 1998): 64–111.

Reinhardt, Uwe. "Wanted—A Clearly Articulated Social Ethic for American Healthcare." *Journal of the Medical American Association* 278 (November 5, 1997): 1446–47.

Rhodes, Robert P. *Health Care, Politics, Policy, and Distributive Justice: The Ironic Triumph.* Albany: State University of New York, 1992.

Rodwin, Marc A. *Medicine, Money & Morals, Physicians' Conflicts of Interest.* New York: Oxford University Press, 1993.

Rothman, David J. *Strangers at the Bedside.* New York: Basic Books, 1991.

Russell, Louise, "The Role of Prevention in Health Reform." *New England Journal of Medicine* 329 (July 29, 1993): 352–54.

Samuelson, Robert J. "The Backlash against HMOs." *Newsweek* (March 9, 1998): 46.

Schorr, Burt "Giving Seniors Better Care without Burdening Doctors." *Physician's Management* (February 1998): 49–54.

Shortell, Stephen, et al. *Remaking Health Care in America.* San Francisco: Jossey-Bass Publishers, 1996.

Spragins, Ellen E. "The Numbers Racket." *Newsweek* (May 5, 1997): 77.

Starr, Paul. *The Logic of Health Care Reform.* New York: Penguin, 1994.

———. *The Social Transformation of American Medicine.* New York: Basic Books, 1982.

Stein, Ruth E. K. *Health Care for Children: What's Right, What's Wrong, What's Next.* New York: United Hospital Fund, 1997.

Strosberg, Martin, et al. *Rationing America's Medical Care: The Oregon Plan and Beyond.* Washington, D.C.: The Brookings Institute, 1992.

Thurston, Jeffrey M. *Death of Compassion: The Endangered Doctor-Patient Relationship.* Waco, Tex.: WRS, 1996.

Tomes, Jonathan P. *Healthcare Privacy & Confidentiality: The Complete Legal Guide*. New York: Irwin Professional Publishing, 1994.

Weissmann, Gerald. *The Doctor Dilemma: Squaring the Old Values with the New Economy*. New York: The Grand Rounds Press, Whittle Direct Books, 1992.

White House Domestic Policy Council. *Health Security, The President's Report to the American People*. New York: Touchstone Books, Simon & Schuster, 1993.

Wilson, Barbara Alden. "Is the Oregon Health Plan Working?" *Unique Opportunities* (January 1996): 32–39.

Wilson, Jennifer Fisher. "Doctors Caught in Prevention Squeeze." *ACP Observer* 18 (February 1998): 1.

Wright, John W., ed. *The New York Times 1998 Almanac*. New York: Penguin, 1997.

Zoloth-Dorfman, Laurie, and Susan Rubin. "The Patient as Commodity: Managed Care and the Question of Ethics." *Journal of Clinical Ethics* 6 (Winter 1995): 339–57.

USEFUL WEBSITES

Ad Hoc Committee to Defend Health Care: http://www.defendhealthcare.org/

Agency for Health Care Policy and Research: http://www.ahcpr.gov/ or http://www.aarp.org/monthly/managedcare/whatismc.html

American Medical Speciality Organization (AMSO) Ethics of Managed Care Forum: http://www.amso.com/ethics.html

Association of American Physicians and Surgeons: http://www2.misnet.com/~rick/pages/purpose.html

Center for Medical Ethics and Health Policy: http://www.bcm.tmc.edu/ethics/

Center for Patient Advocacy: http://www.patientadvocacy.org/main/index.html

Cornell University: http://trochim.human.cornell.edu/gallery/blakesle/cornell.htm

Department of Healthcare Advocacy: http://www.hcp.med.harvard.edu/

Families USA: http://epn.org/families/farisk.html

Fight Managed Care: http://www.his.com/~pico/orgs.htm

Health Care Financial Assistance—The Medicare and Medicaid Agency: http://www.hcfa.gov/

Health Care Liability Alliance: http://www.wp.com/hcla

Health Insurance Association of America: http://www.hiaa.org/consumerinfo/index.html

Henry J. Kaiser Family Foundation Link Library: http://www.kff.org/links/linkhp.html

HMO Page: http://www.hmopage.com/

Institute for Philosophy and Public Policy: http://www.puaf.umd.edu/ippp/

Internet Health Resources: http://www.ihr.com/

Johns Hopkins University Health Information: http://www.intelihealth.com/

Joint Commission on Accreditation of Health Care Organizations: http://www.jcaho.org/

Links to Health Care Websites: http://www.jcaho.org/link_frm.htm

Managed Care Magazine: http://www.managedcaremag.com/

Managed Care Resources, University of Medicine and Dentistry, New Jersey: http://www.umdnj.edu/others/Managed.html

MCARE: http://www.mcare.net/index.html

Medicaid and Managed Care Resource Center: http://www.chcs.org/CHCS/resource.htm

Medicare-Medicaid Statistics and Data: http://www.hcfa.gov/stats/stats.htm

MedWeb Bioethics: http://www.gen.emory.edu/medweb/medweb.bioethics.html

National Center for Health Statistics: http://www.cdc.gov/nchswww/index.htm

National Center for Policy Analysis: www.public-policy.org/~ncpa/pi/health/hedex.html

National Coalition on Health Care: http://www.americashealth.org/

National Committee for Quality Assurance: http://www.ncqa.org/

National Health Information Center: http://nhic-nt.health.org/#Referrals

National Organization of Physicians Who Care: http://www.pwc.org/index.html

RAND Health: http://www.rand.org/organization/health/

Urban Institute: http://www.urban.org/

U.S. Congress on the Internet: http://thomas.loc.gov/

U.S. Department of Health and Human Services: http://www.os.dhhs.gov/

Vote Smart: http://www.votesmart.org/issues/Immigration/chap2/imm2b.htm

William M. Mercer Health and Group Benefits: http://www.mercer.com/hr/Providing_Health_and_Group_Benefits.html

About the Author

Michael E. Makover, M.D., has been assistant professor of Clinical Medicine and Attending at the New York University Medical Center since 1980. He is in private practice, specializing in internal medicine and rheumatology. He was previously on the faculty of Cornell Medical School in both medicine and public health.

Professor Makover received his bachelor's degree from The Johns Hopkins University, where he was elected to Phi Beta Kappa, and his M.D. degree from the Columbia University College of Physicians and Surgeons. He did postgraduate training in internal medicine at The Thomas Jefferson University Hospital in Philadelphia and Mount Sinai Hospital in New York. He then completed fellowships in rheumatology (arthritis and related disorders) at the Hospital for Special Surgery in New York and at the University of California, San Francisco.

He is a Diplomate of the American Board of Internal Medicine, a fellow of the New York Academy of Medicine and the American College of Rheumatology, and a member of the American College of Physicians and other medical societies.

His medical career has spanned an unusually broad spectrum. While primarily in solo private practice, he is experienced in three specialties—internal medicine, rheumatology, and public health—and has worked in and studied medical care in every kind of setting. He has taught in medical school, done research, cared for both wealthy and disadvantaged patients, and knows the corporate world. He was a research associate on Senator Robert Kennedy's staff, where he met the senator and worked on areas of health for possible political action. Dr. Makover also served as a spokesperson for the New York City divisions of the American Cancer Society and the American Heart Association.

He is the author of an article on Lyme disease for *New York Magazine* ("Tick, Tick, Tick") and the foreword to *Free Money for Diseases on Aging,* by Laurie Blum.

Dr. Makover lives near New York City with his wife and two children. He enjoys tennis, reading, photography, and the computer.

Index

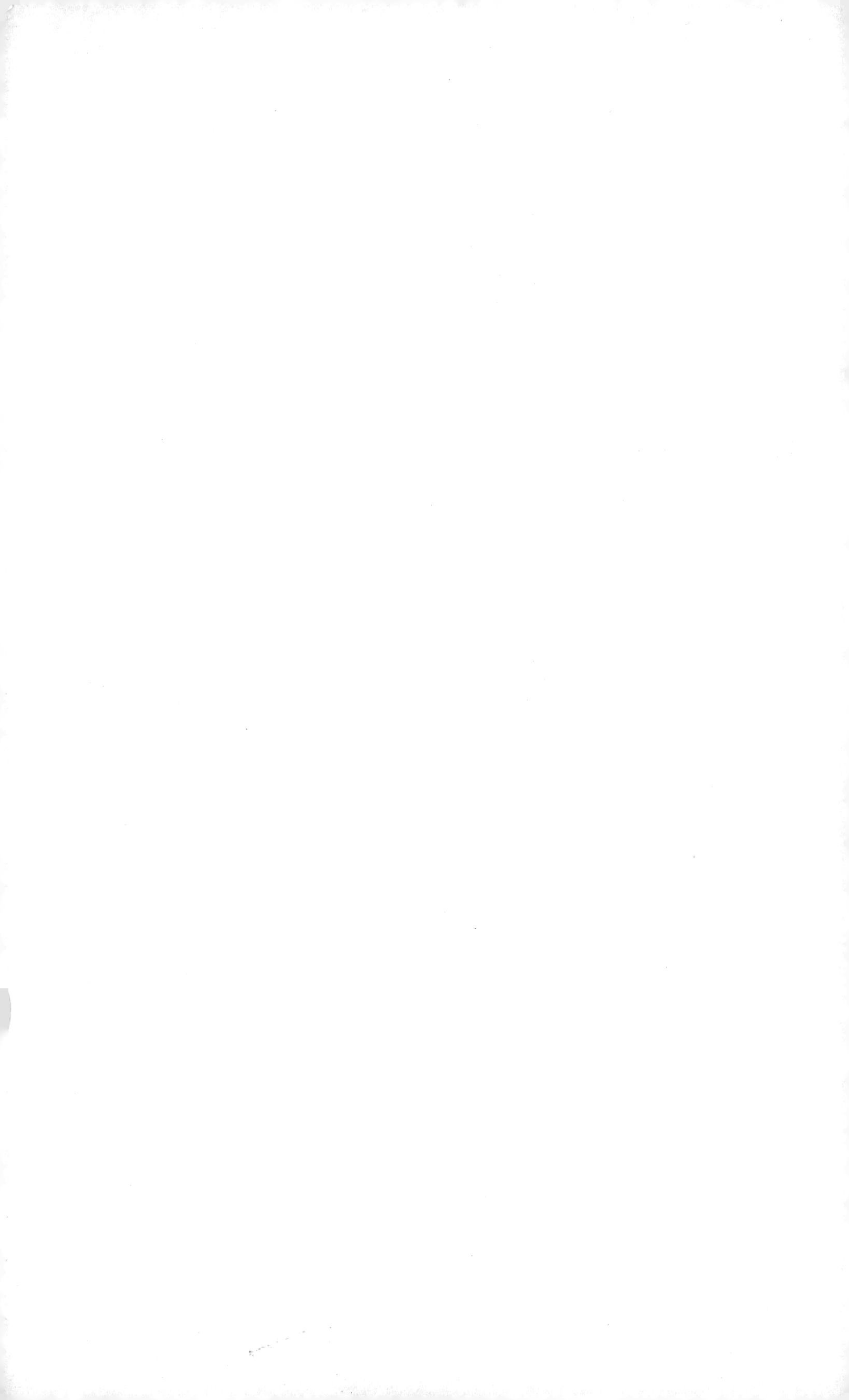